HYPNOSIS FOR LOVERS...
2ND EDITION

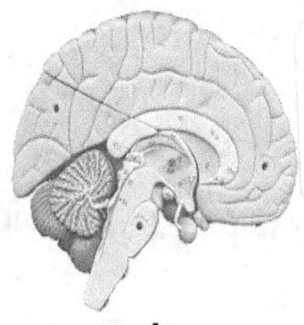

^

SEX ORIGINATES HERE
NOT BETWEEN YOUR LEGS

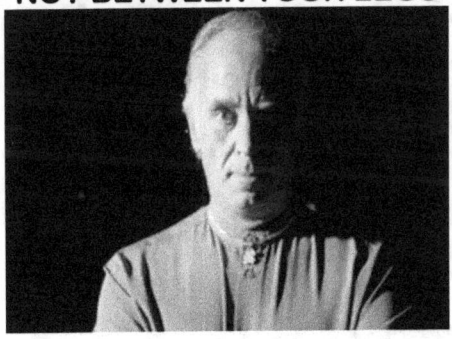

Richard Anthony

STAGE HYPNOTIST, LECTURER & AUTHOR

CONTENTS

ACKNOWLEDGEMENTS

To: Grey's Anatomy & Web MD for the Charts Herein

To: Justin Tranz & Laurie Handlers for Their Support and Assistance

DEDICATION

To All The People Past & Present Who Have Made My 40+ Years In The Hypnosis Field A Joy. Both On Stage & In The Trainings...Thank You All

PREFACE:
ABOUT THE AUTHOR

Hypnotic Greetings:

For over 40 years I've been a hypnotist both stage and therapeutic. In 1968 shortly before my 21st birthday, I had met a stage hypnotist who I ended up having a thirteen year relationship with not only because she was a gorgeous blonde, but also because she cured me of my "disease" through hypno-sex. Here is the short version of that story:

When I was in my mid teens my Dad came into the bathroom when I was actually in the bathtub to teach me about the "birds and the bees". It was embarrassing to say the least because who wants to talk about sex with your Father when you are naked in the tub. Not to mention I was almost 16 years old so he got to me a little late. Anyway at the end of the lecture as it was, he said to me; "I hope you didn't inherit my disease". Of course I asked what his "disease" was and he said in an embarrassed way; "Premature Ejaculation". He went on to explain what it was.

I was a late bloomer and it wasn't until I was 19 and in the USAF when I was first with a woman for sex. Well my first 3 times I could not last, longer than a few seconds (Naturally) so I was convinced I had "The Disease".

I was transferred to Nellis AFB in Las Vegas in 1969 and it was there I went to see a hypnosis show at the Tropicana and ended up on stage. After the show, the female hypnotist sent her manager to invite me backstage. She floored me by telling me we had been lovers in a "past life" But hell she was gorgeous...so I was up (literally) for whatever she wanted to tell me. I ended up going out for drinks with her after about an hour's conversation about reincarnation. It seemed she was interested in me and invited me back to her hotel room. After kissing and petting, she suggested going to the bed. I said to her "I can't"..."I have a disease." A concerned look came over her face and she asked why I had not gone to the base hospital for a treatment to cure it. I told her I had inherited it and it was incurable. She got me almost to tears as I told her what my "disease" was. (You should be chuckling at this point...She was.) To make a long story short she hypnotized me and made love to me...Holding off my climax until she was there with me, a good 20 minutes later. From that point on, my "disease" disappeared and the techniques you are about to read and learn are the result of 40 plus years of research and the study of hypnosis in various aspects. In this book, you will benefit from that knowledge and realize what can be done with hypnosis in the bedroom and many other locations of your choice and imagination.

SEGMENT 1. GETTING TO KNOW HYPNOSIS:

PREFACE: All Hypnosis Is Self-Hypnosis (Not Exactly True)

As you have probably seen, there is so much misinformation out there about hypnosis, that it is no wonder it has the reputation of being so strange and mysterious. In actuality, it is a totally normal brain function that everyone with few exceptions, experiences daily in his or her lives.

In fact, for a long time, there was a debate in scientific circles as to whether or not Hypnosis actually existed. But in 1998, Duke University put the question to rest. They did an intensive year long study, using the latest CAT scan technology, and proved beyond a doubt that the brain chemistry of a hypnotized person is significantly altered when they achieve a hypnotic state.

But what exactly is hypnosis? Well hypnotists say that "all hypnosis self-hypnosis". So let's look at that statement, and try to differentiate between the two common forms of self-hypnosis that each of you could and probably would experience:

The first is actually unintentional. It can happen to you driving in your car, and suddenly realizing that you've been on a sort of "automatic pilot" for several miles. Or becoming engrossed in a good book, or TV show and not realizing what is going on around you. Maybe even not feeling how much time has passed. And of course we all know the most common of all, the daydream, which is simply the time during the day, when your mind wanders off. All of these states are natural shifts in your brain waves.

But the second forms are intentional. Self-Hypnosis, Meditation, Yoga, Chanting, and other mind quieting and focusing practices are all ways in which we can shift the human mind to that altered consciousness "daydreaming state" with one difference. We are actually directing that "daydream". This is accomplished by relaxing your body with internalized suggestions. You have to find a quiet comfortable place, and begin relaxing your muscle groups one by one, then suggesting to your mind that it also relax at the same time. As the mind and body relax, you can actually feel the shift as your body functions slow. It has been likened to the feeling you get just before you fall asleep. Bear in mind that actually hypnosis is **NOT** a technique...It is a state of mind that is quite different from normal sleep. The hypnotic state is actually a very heightened state of consciousness in which one is able to affect and reprogram certain behaviors and body functions. Once you have achieved this state, your "critical mind", the portion that examines and makes judgments about everything you do, is set off to the side, and you are more open to new ideas, suggestions, and concepts. Your sub-conscious mind is now more in charge. It is very much like a computer. It accepts inputs without judgments. This is the basic "why and how" of hypnotic suggestion. But now let's examine what hypnosis or self-hypnosis can and can't do, and what will and won't work:

First and foremost, hypnosis is not magic. No one can wave their hand or perhaps stare into your eyes and sap your will, as we often see done in horror or sci-fi movies. It simply doesn't work that way. You can't be turned into a mindless puppet, unless of course that's what you want to be in some deep-seated fantasy.

No one using hypnosis can make you rob a bank, or do something you consider morally wrong. When you see films like "The Manchurian Candidate", bear in mind they are mostly fiction. And what is not fiction is describing a process called brainwashing, in which hypnosis is combined with other psychological and chemical techniques over a long period of time to drastically modify a persons' behavior. That is not the purpose of what you will learn from this HYPNOSIS FOR LOVERS course.
What you will learn is an exciting new way to stimulate your sex life and that of your partner,

using the largest and strongest sex organ in your body...Your own minds! Along with this, we will also suggest to you some physical stimulation to combine with the mental hypnosis aspects to really put some fireworks into your lovemaking.

And while we will teach you self-hypnosis so that you can improve how you approach HYPNOSIS FOR LOVERS, our main objective will be to teach you to hypnotize your sex partner, and vice versa. Why? Well with self-hypnosis you always have a part of your conscious mind working to direct your "self trance". But, when you let your partner help you achieve hypnosis and guide your trance, you can totally let go and achieve deeper levels of both trance and mental and physical stimulation. This is how your lovemaking experience can be forever transformed into heights you didn't think possible.

And finally, for those of you that think learning hypnosis is difficult, you'll quickly learn that it is not that way at all. Everything you need to know to safely and effectively put someone in a hypnotic state of mind is contained here. It takes a bit of practice, but almost anyone can learn to hypnotize, and be hypnotized. In fact the statement that "I can't be hypnotized" is so far from the truth it is almost laughable. As we have told you above, we all enter hypnotic states several times a day. If you are happen not to take this course with your "significant other" then you should learn all the facts above about hypnosis to explain to the person you want to hypnotize for the first time

SO LET'S BEGIN!

CHAPTER 1. HOW TO HYPNOTIZE THE BASICS:

The Pre-Induction & Test:

We often get asked...is hypnosis dangerous? The answer is absolutely not...So long as you are not trying to be a therapist with what we are teaching you. This course is not designed for that purpose. It is designed to teach you and your partner how to enhance your love life with hypnosis. Although, we will also show you how to use it in your everyday life to make improvements such as motivation, overcoming bad habits, and self improvement, we strongly advise you not to attempt any type of therapy with it without proper further study into the therapeutic aspects of hypnosis.

And while everyone can be hypnotized at some time or other (Unless you have an IQ of less than 50.) some people are better on their first try than others. We're about to show you, and you're about to learn, several ways of determining your HQ (Hypnosis Quotient). These are tests to determine how easily someone can be hypnotized. Normally you would have to build a "rapport" with the person you wanted to hypnotize. But, if you are already in a relationship with someone, the rapport should be "built in". But for teaching purposes, we'll show you how to start from the beginning.

The first test and variation of it to determine just how suggestible the person you want to hypnotize is called a "Hand Clasp Test" & "The Magnetic Fingers Test" respectively. They are simple and easy methods to determine if someone is in the frame of mind to get hypnotized at that particular moment. We will be teaching them to you, and having you practice it on the person you have chosen to hypnotize. As you will see, there are several possibilities that can happen with the test. But again, for teaching purposes, we are going to assume that one of the first two has happened. If you get a really good response and the person's hands are stuck together, then you can congratulate them, and continue on to the induction. If not, but they were somewhat "stuck" then do the second "Sway Test" to further determine their HQ (Hypnosis Quotent).

THE HAND CLASP TEST:

Now that you have established cooperation and trust, you want to bring the person into a soft environment, with a comfortable chair or sofa, and subdued lighting: (In actuality this works anywhere in any type of environment, as we have learned over the years.)

YOU: Just have a seat (or stand) right here, and make yourself as comfortable as you possibly can. Now here's what I want you to do...Fold your hands together in your lap just like this...Good, now I want you to concentrate on your thumbs...Just stare at your thumbs...And begin by taking a nice deep breath just breath in very deeply...And hold it...hold it...exhale and relax...Now take a second deep breath as you continue to stare at your thumbs...And hold it...hold it...exhale and relax...Now I want you to close your eyes...That's right...And imagine that we just put your hands in-between a vise...and that vise is turning down...And as it does...I want you to squeeze your hands together...tighter...and tighter...we're turning it a little more...And you're squeezing tighter...Good, now I want you to imagine that we just opened a can of super glue...and poured it all over your hands...Imagine you can feel it drying ...and on the count of 3...you will find your hands are STUCK & GLUED tight together...And you cannot take them apart...1, 2, & 3...And the harder you try...the tighter they stick...All right...stop trying...open your eyes...and as I touch your hands...they'll totally relax and come apart...

VARIATION ONE: THE MAGNETIC FINGER TEST:

This is very similar to the hand clasp test, but different in the fact that you are dealing with a smaller muscle group. Instead of involving the whole hands and arms, it simply involves the two index fingers of the person, and is a bit easier for you to influence with your suggestions:

YOU: Just have a seat (or stand) right here, and make yourself as comfortable as you possibly can. Now here's what I want you to do; fold your hands together in front of your face. Now, put your index fingers up about two inches apart and begin to stare at them...Take a deep breath now and just relax...Now as you continue to stare at them, you can feel your fingers start to become just like magnets...They are irresistibly drawing together... Just like magnets now...The closer they begin to get...The stronger the pull is...That's right...Feel them closing...See them getting closer and closer together...Their magnetic attraction getting stronger and stronger...And in a few seconds they will touch and be stuck to each other...Just like two super strong magnets...Stuck so tight that you cannot take them apart...That's right... STUCK & GLUED tight together now until I touch and them and de-magnetize them...(You let them try...then touch them.)

That was great... You were incredible...Let's move on...(To an induction.)

(It is important at this point to access the situation) 1. If the person's hands or fingers were totally stuck, then you have an excellent candidate for hypnosis on your hands. 2. If they were somewhat stuck, but the person was starting to take them apart, quickly tell them they are no longer stuck, and do the "Sway Test" to further convince them that they can be hypnotized. If your person falls in to category # 2, then proceed to the second test. If they are in category # 1, then you can proceed right to the hypnotic induction.

THE "FORWARD SWAY TEST":

This second test is very convincing to someone who experiences it. As you will see, it is an involuntary response to your suggestions. Your partners' body will begin to "sway" without any conscious effort on his or her part. Just make sure to plant that foot back so you can support their weight. Often, this test will overcome the doubt in your partners' conscious mind and make it much easier for you to proceed with their first hypnosis session. Later, we'll even teach you how to turn any of these tests into actual hypnotic inductions.

YOU: That was great...I want to just show you one more thing...(Put your hand out to lead them.) Come right up here...Now I want you to put your feet together...and just let your arms hang loose at your side...Just relax and let me do the work... Focus your eyes on mine...(Look at the bridge of their nose, and it will look as though you are looking right through them.)...And I'm going to rock you gently back and forth...just like this (Put your hands firmly on their shoulders and rock them slowly back and forth)...Keep your eyes focused on mine...and when I take my hands away...You'll find that you'll FALL FORWARD... right into my arms...Don't worry...don't even think about it...I'll catch you...(Make sure you are standing solidly with one foot braced behind your other, so that you can support the persons weight.) ... Rocking...NOW...ROCKING...LET GO... YOU KNOW YOU CAN TRUST ME COMPLETELY... (Remove your hands but keep eye contact.) ...FALLING STRAIGHT TO ME...(Keep the falling suggestion going until they are coming onto you...then say) VERY GOOD...YOU ARE GREAT AT THIS.

VARAITION: "THE REVERSE SWAY"

This is done exactly in the same manner as the Forward Sway with the following exception. You will have them close their eyes and tilt their head back as though they are looking at an imaginary spot on the ceiling...And of course you will change your wording to FALLING BACK into my arms...(If they fall in either variation without putting their foot out to balance themselves then they are ready to be hypnotized. If not work with them until they do...What carefully what they are doing when you take them back upright. If they are helping you in any way, make them notice it and tell them to stop it...

Now, it is always a good idea to practice this with someone without trying to get any results and having them just do it with you so you can get the feel of it, and how you should stand to support their body weight. IF THERE IS AN EXTREME DIFFERENCE IN YOUR BODY WEIGHTS...DO NOT ATTEMPT THIS TEST. For example, if you are a female and weigh 125 pounds, do not have a 250 pound man fall on you...It's just not a good idea, especially if you can't support them. But, you can adjust the amount of space between you and the other person so that they don't fall far enough to have and significant impact on you when they fall.

YOUR FIRST HYPNOTIC INDUCTION

FRACTIONAL RELAXATION:

This is one of the most tried and true inductions used in traditional hypnosis (You will be learning Ericksonian and what I call the TRANZ methods after my friend Justin Tranz who developed them a bit later.) It involves relaxing all the muscle groups in your partners' body to lead them into trance, then deepening that trance with suggestions. Below is the actual script, so you can follow along. Once again, you will want to use a couch or comfortable chair. If you have a recliner, that's even better, and bring a second chair so that you can sit next to the person.

YOU: I want you to just sit back relax and focus your eyes on the light...Do not take your eyes away off that light...Make yourself as comfortable as possible, but do not cross your legs, or clasp your hands, so that your circulation can flow freely...Now I want you to start by again taking a nice deep breath...Just breathe in deeply...and hold it...Hold it...Exhale and relax...Now take a second deep breath a little deeper this time...And hold it...Hold it...Exhale and relax...Now one last time...A nice deep deep breath...And hold it...Hold it...Exhale and relax...

(WHAT YOU JUST DID WAS OVER OXYGENATE THEIR BODY WHICH WILL CAUSE A SLIGHT DIZZY OR TINGLING FEELING IN THEIR BODY, RESULTING IN THEIR CONSCIOUS MIND FEELING SOMETHING IS HAPPENING.)

I'm going to count backwards from ten to 0...On the count of 0 I want you to close your eyes...Now you may feel like closing your eyes before I get to 0...If you do that's fine...But if you do not...on the count of 0 I want you to close your eyes...TEN...Begin to relax every muscle in your entire body...Just let go...let go completely... NINE...Complete and total relaxation should be your only goal now...EIGHT...Relaxing more and more completely...more and more deeply... with every word I say...With every breath you take... SEVEN...You'll find that your eyes are beginning to get heavy...Very very heavy...SIX...Eyes becoming heavier and heavier...Much much heavier...FIVE ..Just let go...Every muscle ... every tendon...every cell in your body...FOUR...Relaxing deeper and deeper down now...with every word that I say...with every breath you take...THREE...Your eyes are so heavy now heavier and heavier...and your whole body is just becoming so relaxed ...TWO...Your eyes are so heavy now...so very heavy that you want to close your eyes...ONE & ZERO...close your eyes now...close your eyes and relax.

(What you should be looking for during this 10 count is the persons' eyelids beginning to flutter and close...and their breathing starting to become rhythmic.)

YOU: Now I want you to start with your left foot...and withdraw all the muscle power in your left foot...Just let go...Let go completely...Now let this nice warm pleasant relaxation flow and extend up through your ankle...And spread through your calf...Now up over your knee...And up into your thigh...And up into your left hip...So that from your hip to your toe...all the tension is gone...Now let it flow through your right foot...Up through the right ankle...up over your right knee

...and into your right thigh...Up through your right hip...and around through your pelvis area...so that the whole bottom half of your body is very warm...very comfortable...and very relaxed...Now I want you to let this wonderful relaxation flow and extend...coming up through the muscles in the small of your back...Relax all the muscles in the small of your back...and let it flow to those large muscles in your upper back...Just let go...Let go completely...Now let it flow on up into your shoulders...Take one more deep breath and as you let it out...collapse your shoulders ...Relax and collapse your shoulders...and let it flow down through your chest...into your abdomen...and particularly the muscles in your stomach...Now I want you to concentrate on relaxing all the muscles in your stomach...Once again just let go...Let go completely ...Now let this nice warm relaxation flow back up through your chest...into your shoulders...and down the muscles of your left arm...From your shoulder to your elbow ...From your elbow to your fingertips...and out the fingertips of your left arm...Now back up into your shoulders...and down your right arm...From your shoulder to your elbow...From your elbow to your fingertips...and out the fingertips of your right arm...Now back up through your shoulders...and I want you to relax all the muscles in your neck...Relax all the muscles in your neck...and let your head fall into a nice comfortable position...Again just let go...Let go completely

...Now let the relaxation flow and extend coming up over your scalp...and spreading down across your face...your forehead...your eyes...your nose... and your mouth...So that from the top of your head...to the bottom of your feet...you are so heavy...so comfortable...and so relaxed...And with each and every word I say... And each and every breath you take...You are sinking and going deeper and deeper down...deeper and deeper asleep...I want you to picture yourself at the top of an escalator...It has 10 stairs...I'm going to count backwards from 10 to 0...As I count backwards from 10 to 0...I want you to picture yourself descending the stairs...and just sleep... way...way... down... TEN... NINE... EIGHT... SEVEN...SIX... FIVE...Deeper... Deeper... FOUR... THREE... TWO... ONE... and ZERO...Just SLEEP... Way way down...Continually going deeper... always going deeper...I'm going to touch your hand...and when I do any last tension in your body will disappear...and you'll sink even deeper asleep...(Touch Hand)...You'll find that you're so heavy...so comfortable...and so relaxed...that your eyes in particular are very comfortable and relaxed...They are so heavy...so comfortable...and so relaxed...that they are STUCK AND GLUED tight together...and you cannot take them apart...And the harder you try...the tighter they stick...you may try...but the harder you try...the tighter they stick...all right...stop trying...relax and just go deeper and deeper down...deeper and deeper asleep.

(This was a test to determine if the person was hypnotized. If they were, you should see their eyelids flutter as they tried to open them. We are now going to perform one more test that will determine how far under hypnosis the person is. There are 5 general depth levels running from light trance to the deepest level called somnambulism. Later you will see how to judge the depth level of the person you have hypnotized.)

Now on the count of three...I want you to raise your right arm high in the air over your head...it will feel light as a feather...1, 2, & 3...Now as it rises...it is becoming stiff and rigid...Stiff and rigid as a steel bar...and nothing on Earth will bend it...And the harder you try to bend your arm...the tighter it's going to get...

(At this point you want to touch the persons arm and pay attention during this test to see how stiff the arm is. The stiffer it is, the deeper in hypnosis the person is. Now let's show you some of the things you can do once someone is hypnotized. But first let's get your partner up and functioning. Now pay attention, because even though their eyes will be open, and they will appear to be wide-awake, they will actually still be hypnotized.)

All right stop trying...Your arm is dropping to your side...and as it does...it will send you even deeper asleep...Now on the count of 3, I want you to sit up, open your eyes, and function normally until I say the word SLEEP. When I say the word SLEEP, you will relax back down in the chair, and go right back into the deep relaxed state you are in right now. If you understand, raise your left index finger...Good, 1, 2, & 3...sit up and open your eyes. How do you feel?

(At this point, you have hypnotized your partner.)

CHAPTER 2: ONCE THEY ARE HYPNOTIZED, THEN WHAT?

The purpose of this course is to teach you how to use hypnosis with your lover. But before we get into that, you can also learn a few things you can do with it outside the bedroom. And it is good practice. It this next chapter, we I'll be showing you how to set up suggestions to improve hand eye coordination in sports. But, their are many other uses and applications. Even if you just want to relieve the tension of a stressful day, 20 minutes with hypnosis can do that easily. So let's show you how this works using a sport as an example...In this case Golf...But it can be adapted to any sport.

YOU: I want you to sit back, relax, and SLEEP...That's right, slipping back down...You told me that you wanted to improve your golf game...and I'm going to show you how easy it is to turn that request over to your sub-conscious mind to process for you. Your sub-conscious mind is actually the largest part of your mind. It controls your breathing...and you don't think about it...It controls your heartbeat...and you don't think about it...And it controls all of the functions of your body...that you never have to think about...Now we're going to turn your golf swing over to it...Every time you step up to the golf ball, whether it's on the tee...the fairway...or the green...your sub-conscious mind will automatically take over your muscle functions, and coordination...Just like it controls your heartbeat...It will give you a perfect coordinated effortless swing, and stroke...In fact we're going to program it into your mind right now...I want you to imagine a smooth strong tee shot...See it in your mind... Feel the coordination of your muscles making a perfect shot...Now let that flow into your sub-conscious and know it will control your tee shots from this point on...Now, I want you to do the same thing with a fairway shot...See it...Now feel the muscles work in harmony ... Now let it flow directly into your sub-conscious...and know your fairway shots will be controlled by your sub-conscious...Now once more with your putts...See them... Let your sub-conscious line up angle of the shot...And see and feel the putt...Now send it...and know your putts will be perfect without having to think or worry about it...From this point on...every time you play a round of golf...your confidence level will be high...Your fears and doubts about difficult shots will not be accepted by your sub-conscious mind. Because it already has the positive programming you just put into it...And just before you step onto the first tee...you'll take a couple of deep breaths to relax your body...and repeat the phrases... "My mind and body have become harmonized ...This harmony will carry through the entire 18 holes of golf...When you do this, it will trigger the sub-conscious programming we just placed in your mind...You will see the effects in your score from the very first time you do this...

(We did this for golf, but as you can well imagine, it works for any sport...And now here is a weight loss scenario you can use.)

You also asked about losing 10 lbs...And just like it will help you improve your golf game...Your subconscious mind will also help you effortlessly lose that ten pounds... When we were in our teens...it was real hard to gain weight...because our metabolism was so high...We were so active that we burned off the calories very quickly...But as we grew older...our metabolism slowed down...However...just like everything else in our bodies ...it is also controlled by that same subconscious mind...So what we're going to do...is turn over your diet to that giant un-conscious that will automatically program your diet for you...I want you to picture yourself traveling deep into your mind's control center...Think of it as a computer...Now, sit down at the keyboard of the computer that the controller of your subconscious mind...Picture yourself opening up the file that says "metabolism"...See how slow it's running...Now type in this command... "For the next three weeks...you will run my metabolism...at the 18 year old rate...And you will link & relay an overwhelming desire to my conscious mind...to eat healthy low fat foods...lots of fruits and vegetables...Small portions of meats...and smaller quantities all around will satisfy my appetite... Walking in the fresh air...or playing more sports activities will be a result of my extra energy from my increased metabolism...Finally...once I shed the ten pounds I am seeking to lose...you will create an overwhelming desire to maintain that weight through a health lifestyle...Now let's proof read it...And now hit ENTER...It asks if this is what you really want to do...YES or NO...Hit YES!...You have just permanently re-programmed your mind to help improve your life... Congratulations!

(We did this for weight reduction, but the same technique can be used for smoking, and other habits...You can also use the same technique to improve memory, work and study habits... almost anything you can come up with, except those things that are caused by real illness, or underlying serious medical or psychological conditions. Remember you are not qualified to practice therapeutic hypnosis. And you can use this segment on yourself with self-hypnosis. Simply read it after you hypnotize yourself with the Fractional Relaxation Method.)

AWAKENING PROCEEDURE:

This is fairly easy, and goes like this:

YOU: on the count of five...I want you totally wide awake...feeling better in mind...and body...and spirit...then you've felt in a long long time...As you know ...one hour of hypnosis is equal to 8 hours sleep...So when you do wake up...you find you have all kinds of energy...Especially that kind of energy I love...

(Yes folks, it works great for that too...But that's a little later, and why you are here reading this.)

And any time in the future that you wish to be hypnotized by me...You'll go easily right back into the same state that you're in right now...By my simply touching your forehead and saying the word SLEEP... (This is a post-hypnotic suggestion, which we will go into shortly.)

But right now, its time for you to be wide-awake...ONE...Start to awaken...TWO... Awakening more and more completely...THREE...Sit up ...and open your eyes... FOUR... more and more awake...And FIVE ...WIDE AWAKE...WIDE AWAKE and FEELING GREAT...(Clap your hands in front of the person.)

Depending on how deep they went, it might take them a couple of minutes to re-orient themselves, just like it does when they wake up in the morning.

POST-HYPNOTIC SUGGESTIONS:

One of the most powerful & useful tools in the practice of hypnosis, is the post-hypnotic suggestion. It allows you to use a key word or phrase to trigger a suggestion you have planted into someone's sub-conscious mind while they are hypnotized. The most common use of this technique is to re-hypnotize someone very quickly, as you can see in this segment below.

YOU: (To your partner who you just woke up) SLEEP, way way down...Right back to the same state you were in!

(It is a good idea to do this right away with someone you have hypnotized for the first time, so that they get used to the feeling. Also, if they have any doubt that you hypnotized them in the first place, this will dispel that doubt.)

YOU: This time when I wake you up, & I say the word_SUMMER, someone turned the heat up in this room. It will get so hot, you'll have to roll up your sleeves or fan yourself, just to cool off...It will stay uncomfortable until I say the word, **NORMAL**, then everything will return to normal, and you will be comfortable again.

It is not necessary for you to remember that I have told you this, you will simply react to the words. On the count of 5, wide awake. (Repeat Awakening Procedure.) Welcome back. How do you feel now? (Wait for their answer.) Great, you know I wanted to tell you that one of my favorite times of the year is <u>SUMMER</u>! I just love the <u>SUMMER</u> (Once they react.) What's the matter? Are you uncomfortable? They will probably say something like: "All of a sudden it got very warm in here." I don't know what you're talking about...I can check if you want, but it feels pretty <u>NORMAL</u> to me. (Watch their reactions now.)

This also shows a form of "temporary amnesia", which can be induced through hypnosis, when you are using a post-hypnotic type suggestion. If you tell someone not to remember, often they will fight through it, but if you suggest that it is "not important to remember" it is more effective.

Now, let's go through a few of the uses of hypnosis that are not medical in nature, and that anyone can practice.

HYPNOSIS & SELF HYPNOSIS:

You have already seen how to give a suggestion for weight reduction, and sports, now lets go through some of the other things you can do with this process. We're going to assume that you have already gone through the induction process.
YOU: You have expressed a strong desire to quit

smoking, and as you continue to relax, that desire is getting so strong, that you will know that this will succeed and you will no longer be a smoker. Part of your habit is a physical addiction to nicotine. It takes place in your brain...And right now, we are going to disconnect that physical craving...I want you to imagine that we have entered the control center of your brain again...Remember, it looks like a giant computer with a keyboard station...Now imagine that you are sitting back at that keyboard...Type in SEARCH...Now type in "nicotine addiction"...As you know...your sub-conscious mind functions just like a big computer ...It will find the center of that addiction quite easily...all right, the center is right there on the screen of your imagination...Now type in the following command...DELETE AND ERASE NICOTINE ADDICTION...Now press ENTER ...It says "CONFIRM DELETE"...Hit YES ...

Now take a deep breath as you feel your brain disconnecting the addiction...Now I want you to again type in SEARCH...And this time type in HABIT CHANGE...See the file open...Now I want you to type in...REPLACE CIGARETTS WITH EXERCISE AND NEW HOBBIES...Now hit ENTER ...And see in your mind...all of the habit and desire for cigarettes being replaced by a desire for a healthy body...and fun new activities...Instead of reaching for a cigarette...You'll find yourself doing stretching & breathing exercises at home, in the office, or the car...Brisk walking if you are outside ...Dancing if you are out for the evening...From this point on...during the next seven days...your mind is disconnecting all the old smoking pathways...Even if you falter...your sub-conscious mind will automatically notice when and why... and immediately fix the faulty input...So that at the end of seven days...you have not only become a proud non-smoker from day one, but also...your appetite...and desire for food will remain just the same...or even decrease as you get healthier ...And your energy level will rise...until it reaches your body's full potential...Picture all this...And once more hit ENTER...Now ENCRYPT the new program, so that it can never change back...Raise your left index finger when you have finished... (Once you see the finger raise, begin the awakening procedure) Congratulations!...And on the count of five, I want you wide awake knowing that from today on...you will be a non-smoker...1 start to awaken...2 awakening more and more completely ...3 sit up and open your eyes...4 more and more awake...and 5 wide awake...wide awake...feeling marvelous...and 5...wide awake feeling great.

Now you have seen two ways to reprogram a persons' sub-conscious inner mind...and implant post-hypnotic suggestions...What can you use it for? The list is endless. But here are a few of the most common uses:

You can stop nail biting...
Overcome the fear of flying...
Lose the fear of public speaking...
Lose the fear of heights...
Improve your memory and organizational skills...
Increase your confidence...
And many more simple behaviors...
Any fear or phobia that is not tied to a deep rooted mental illness responds very well to hypnosis...And you can use any of these on yourself with self-hypnosis...OK, lets show you some different ways and methods to hypnotize different types of people.

CHAPTER 3: DIFFERENT HYPNOTIC TECHNIQUES:

Once you become proficient in the "Fractional Relaxation" method, which is the "catch all" of hypnosis inductions. But now we are going to expand your "Induction Knowledge" So let's start with one of the most useful ones...When you attempt to do hypnosis you are going to come across certain people with an analytical personality...Often, they have analytical jobs such as an accountant for example...And quite often they are a bit difficult to hypnotize...because they are to busy trying to figure out what is happening instead of letting themselves relax...For this type of person...a distraction method often works best. You must give their conscious mind a monotonous analytical type task to perform, while you are implanting suggestions into their sub-conscious mind...You will be expanding your knowledge to other inductions as we proceed in this chapter.

1. DISTRACTION METHOD

(Let's call our friend JOHN for the purpose of this script. We will also assume that you have had a pre-induction talk with them and they are willing to try.)

John, I'd like you to have a seat (or stand) right over here...and make yourself as comfortable as you possibly can...Now focus your eyes on mine...and I'd like you to do this for me...Count backwards from 100...and after each two counts count...say the words "Deep Sleep" for me...I'm going to talk to you while you're counting, but I don't want you to worry about what I'm saying...I just want you to concentrate on counting...OK? (Get a yes so you know they understand.)...Let's begin...

(Get close to the person and begin talking in a slow, rhythmic, soft, but firm voice.)

...*100 deep sleep...99 deep sleep...*Yes, your mind is becoming focused on a deep and restful sleep...*98 deep sleep...97 deep sleep...* your body beginning to relax now...Getting ready for deep sleep...*96 deep sleep ...95 deep sleep...*Your breathing slow and steady now...your counting slower now as you relax...*94 deep sleep...93 deep sleep...* Your eyes are relaxing now...Beginning to get heavy...*92 deep sleep ...91 deep sleep...*Your eyes are so heavy now...Your whole body becoming limp, loose, and relaxed...*90 deep sleep...89 deep sleep...* your eyes are too heavy to keep open...On the next count they close...*88 deep sleep ...87...deep sleep*

(At this point, if the persons eyes are closed you can proceed as follows, if not keep them counting, and keep suggesting heavier and heavier eyelids, until they close, then proceed.

They will very rarely get past 80.)

Eyes heavy and closed now...so relaxed that counting is no longer important...*86 deep sleep...85 deep sleep*...I'll take over counting...so that you can get that DEEP SLEEP... 84...(Here just start with the fractional relaxation as you count.) Start with your feet...and withdraw every bit of muscle power from your feet ...83 Now let this nice comfortable relaxation flow and extend...

(Once you have done their whole body, stop counting and proceed with the escalator deepening starting a count at ten to zero.)

2. HAND CLASP/MAGNET FINGERS TO HYPNOSIS:

This method is a very fast way to hypnotize a large percent-age of the people you come across who react well to your Hand Clasp or Magnetic Fingers Test. It is simple to do and very effective. You simply go from your final statement where their hands (or fingers) are stuck and glued to this without un-sticking them:

YOU: (As you push down sharply on their hands which are still stuck, with one hand and their head with the other from the back...at the same time, and slowly lay them on the floor.) SLEEP...THE HARDER YOU TRY TO PULL YOUR HANDS (fingers) APART THE DEEPER YOU GO NOW...Deeper and deeper down with every count you hear me say...TEN...Begin to relax every muscle in your entire body...Just let go...let go completely...NINE...Complete and total relaxation should be your only goal now...EIGHT...Relaxing more and more completely...more and more deeply... with every word I say...With every breath you take... SEVEN...You'll find that you are sinking and beginning to get heavy...Very very heavy ...SIX...Your entire body becoming heavier and heavier...Much much heavier...FIVE...Just let go... Every muscle...every tendon...every cell in your body...FOUR...Relaxing deeper and deeper down now...with every word that I say...with every breath you take...THREE ... You are so heavy now heavier and heavier...and your whole body is just becoming so relaxed...TWO...You are so heavy now...so very heavy and slipping and sliding deeper and deeper...ONE & ZERO...Deep Deep Sleep Now...

(You can continue to deepen them with suggestions or refer back to the Fractional Relaxation Induction to continue to relax muscle groups one at a time.)

If you remember back to our first hand-clasp test, we showed you how to perform a second "sway test" with a person that was questionable. However, you can also use a variation of that test with a person who is not questionable, but rather passed the hand-clasp test with flying colors. In other words, their hands were stuck together very tightly. After the hand-clasp test, compliment the person and tell them they are doing a great job of relaxing and following directions.

THE JUSTIN TRANZ EYELOCK METHOD

One of my oldest friends and fellow hypnotists in Las Vegas is Justin Tranz: Over the years, I have come to admire and now use almost exclusively his induction method, which he adapted from both Dave Elman, and Milton Erickson with a bit of the techniques of Richard Bandler thrown in and then combined with his own unique perspective. What I am about to share with you, you can see on YOU TUBE: https://www.youtube.com/watch?v=zmh4uZJQXEg So that you can get an exact idea of how it works.

LEAD IN: Stand right in front of me...and put your feet together...Make them touch, and do not move your feet. In a moment, I'm going to rock you slightly off balance...Just go where I put you, I've got you...I want you to just keep your eyes focused on mine... That's right...Now just put yourself in my hands as I start to rock your body slowly back and forth...Back and forth...(This is the forward sway portion where you put your hands on their shoulders to get them started and rock them forward...till they start to fall forward...If they put their foot out make them notice they did that, and start over saying: I will not let you fall...I'VE GOT YOU...) Once they fall forward then move around in back of them and do a sway backward in the same manner. Then stand in front of them, looking at them and say: FEEL THIS as you make a slight movement to one side or the other...But be ready to move fast and support them in any direction they sway. After you get a movement and put them back upright, take a step back after raising both their arms slightly and lightly slapping them back to their sides and once again look at them...this time focusing on their hands saying: NOW FEEL THIS...(Looking from one hand to the next till you see movement... Then whichever moves focus on it and work on them raising it: THAT'S RIGHT...MMM HMM MORE HIGHER...ETC. Once it raises even a little...call their attention to it: WATCH IT...THAT'S RIGHT IT'S CRAZY ISN'T IT?...Then from here go right into the EYELOCK pictured in the YOUTUBE video.

NLP & INSTANT INDUCTIONS:

We are just going to touch briefly on this...And more for your knowledge than actual instruction, because learning these methods is better left to "hands on" or video instructions, which I will tell you how to get at the end of the course here.

NLP refers to Neuro Linguistic Programming. If you have ever heard the term that "Words Have

Power" it fits NLP perfectly. Basically, the way the human brain is wired, it reacts to some language patterns far more than others. A hypnotic researcher named Milton Erickson did life long research into it and his legacy is called Ericksonian Hypnosis. Richard Bandler and John Grindler picked up the torch after he passed away and refined Ericksonian Hypnosis into Neuro Linguistic Programming. Below is a simple example of it for your perusal done in a poetic style developed by my friend JoAnne with some edits and additions by me (Richard Anthony):

POETIC NLP

Hello, I'm working on something I need an opinion from you on. You'll do that for me won't you? (You want to get a Yes Response at least 2 times.)
(Yes)
Well it's an attempt at a new form of poetry called "Sensory Poetry" You need to feel it as well as listen to it. I knew you'd be just the right person to be able to do that...Don't you agree?
(Yes)
Great...Get comfy...and listen carefully:

In your mind you feel the swirling thoughts sometimes.
The ones that often make it hard to focus...to unwind.

Feel them now...like windmills...circling round and round

Flowing like a cyclone...but never quite touching down

They're often confusing...like scattered leaves in the wind

Try to focus on one...and a hundred others come rushing in

Grab one now...perhaps a tidbit from your busy day...

The others rush in on you...that thought just flies away

Replaced by another wanting your complete attention

That upon examination...is hardly worth the mention

Thoughts upon thoughts...slipping in...and sliding out

So jumbled sometimes...you don't know what they're about

So much nicer don't you think...not to have to think

To listen to pleasant rhymes....link upon soothing link

My voice link into your ears...directly to your mind

Settling in so deeply....Soon helping you unwind.

Even as your conscious thoughts continue to slip and stray
Feel a deeper part...now focusing totally...on what I say
Pleasant rushing streams and warm tendrils of my voice
Seeping deep inside you...let them in now by your choice

Enveloping you with waves of the most pleasant feelings
Other thoughts are simply leaving...as you feel our mind bonds sealing
Notice how my voice can sweep your cares away
Listen even closer now...Lock on to what I say...

Isn't it interesting...you're floating down on my words
So melodic...so enticing...resistance is absurd
Feel you mind shifting now...bonding with mine
So pleasant to let go now...to totally unwind...

As you slip and slide down on my poetic words...
The last of your resistance floats off like a bird
You trance deep...floating softly to the bottom...
Is it Winter...Spring...Summer...or Autumn?

Thoughts flowing in and out over and around...
Swirling...circling being pulled deeply down
You're enveloped now in my poem of sleep...
Forever melting for me...Forever slipping deep.

NLP....Here is a basic "primer" into how to use NLP words and phrases:

THE 18 MOST POWERFUL WORDS

1. Naturally
2. Easily   Adverb/Adjective
3. Unlimited

4. Aware
5. Realize(ing)   Awareness
6. Experience(ing)

7. Before
8. During   Time / Number
9. After

10. Among
11. Expand   Spatial
12. Beyond

13. And
14. As   Cause and Effect
15 Causes

16. Because
17. Now   Commands
18. Stop

First, you'll note that the words are grouped into 6 sections. In each section, you'll note the category name to the right. I have chosen several of the most powerful examples of each of the categories to make up the 18 most powerful words for persuasion.

Strategy for using Adverb/Adjective Presuppositions:

ALWAYS put Adverbs before the verb and Adjectives before the noun.
1. Naturally
2. Easily
3. Unlimited
MAJOR NOTE: Everything that follows one of these words is pre-supposed in the sentence. In other words, you have to accept everything that follows as true in order to make sense of the sentence.

Examples:
1. Have you discovered how *easily* you can make the decision to refer your friends to our company?
2. Have you asked yourself if the *unlimited* potential of this information is what is making you so excited?
3. Have you naturally discovered how persuasive you are becoming?
4 Many people begin *naturally*, Mr. Williams to create an idea of owning this just prior to making the decision to go ahead with it.
5. Naturally, you'll find more than enough reasons to go ahead today if you understand even a little

bit of what I say next.

REMEMBER - put the words that describe, in front of what they're describing. This forces powerful pictures in the mind of the listener. This is not only powerful and effective in speaking, it's also very effective in writing copy.

The 3 words that you have been given in the Adverb/Adjective category are, as you have probably figured out by now, representative of a whole class of descriptive type words that will have this same type of impact when you use them. I gave you the most important 3 that I use on a regular basis. Here's a bigger list that you can also choose from:
Some all many begin easily naturally
readily infinife(ly) unlimited continue begin still already repeatedly usually finally most truly immediately
Pack as many of these words as possible together without sounding (too) strange!
Examples:
1. You've probably started to become aware of *some* of the *many easily* yet *powerful* ways you can use this information
2. *Naturally,* the *most readily* available and *more importantly, competent* person to deal with is me.
3. *Finally,* the *most reliably accurate system* of persuasion is within your grasp.

Here's a power packed one for you:

Have you asked yourself recently how many services your present broker (or whomever) should be providing, but is not? (pause) Since, I brought that up, does it make you wonder how much more you could be getting when we do your investing (or whatever)?

When you use these patterns in writing, don't pack them together to hard or it will make your writing unclear. In speaking, pack them in as much as possible.

Now we move on to the Most Powerful Words. 4, 5, and 6 -
4. Aware
5. Realize(ing)
6. Experience(ing)
This is the Awareness category.
This is one of my personal favorites because simply saying one of these words, makes the person you are persuading, start to do the mental process that you brought up.
These words are very important to your persuasion arsenal because, like the Adverb/Adjective words, everything that follows them is presupposed to be true. Also, these words force the issue of not will you do X (whatever you suggest), but are you aware that X.
By the way, as you gain skill in using these words,

this scenario will never happen, however, if it does - here's what to do. Let's say you ask the question, "Are you aware that ... ." and the person you're persuading says, NO. You simply respond with, "OH, not yet, huh?! "

Examples:
1. Is the *awareness* of the power of these patterns starting to sink in?
2. The more you begin to construct in your mind the ways you'll be using these patterns after you return home, the more you' ll begin *realizing* the explosively profitable techniques you now possess.
3. Are you starting to *experience* the satisfaction of what owning this will bring as I tell you about it?
And of course, you can combine them just like the others to create super-powered suggestions.
4. Becoming *aware* of the potentials of this policy allows you to start *experiencing* the inner sense of *realizing* how completely this program fits your needs.
Of course, you can also combine these words with the Adverb/Adjective group of words for even more impact.

Remember no pattern is an island! Strength comes from combining as many patterns together as possible.
Here's an example:

5. *Naturally*, as you start *realizing* the *unlimited ways* you can *easily* become *aware* of how joining this team will help you to *truly* accomplish your goals more *rapidly* and *effectively*, you'll start *imagining* the success you can *actually* achieve with my help
and guidance - *NOW* - are you starting to experience the possibilities?

Of course, as before, the words I choose are my personal favorites. Here are some additional words in this category that you can also choose from:
realize(ing) aware know understand(ing)
think(ing) feel(ing) wonder(ing) puzzle(ing)
speculate(ing) perceive(ing) discover(ing)
experience(ing)
accomplish(ing) fulfill(ing) grasp(ing)
reconsider(ing)
weigh(ing) consider assume(ing) conceive(ing)

Now we move on to the Most Powerful Words, 7, 8 and 9 -
7. Before
8. During
9. After
This is the Time/Number category.
These words use some aspect of Time and or Numbers to create the presuppositions of your choice. It is very difficult to distinguish between Time and Number as categories so they are

combined. The easiest way to define this category, is to give some examples.

1. *After* you work with me you'll understand.

2. *Before* you decide just how easy this decision is to make, let me tell you a few things that might help, o.k.?

3. *During* our time together today, could you be applying the benefits you will be discovering about this (product or service) to your life?

And of course, you can combine all the patterns together to get even more exciting suggestions -

4. *During* our discussion today, *naturally*, you'll begin *experiencing* excitement about what the future holds for you as you *begin* to *understand* how *easily* this information is for you.

Here's a larger list of words that fit into this category as well for you to use:

Before, former, was, currently, while

During, after, when, foremost, continue

Earlier, later, until, firstly, eventually

Secondly, highest, foremost, other, in addition to

Chief, another, earliest, latest, more

Now we move on to the Most Powerful Words 10, 11 and 12 -

10. Among

11. Expand

12. Beyond

This is the Spatial category.

Spatial words are always used to create some relationship between things. This could be

hypnotic thought, ideas, products, services or
These words evoke powerful imagery in the mind
of the listener as well.

Here are some examples:

1. From *among* the positive thoughts that you're already starting to realize you have about working with our firm, will come the most obvious, yet *overlooked* reason to bring us on board now.

(Of course, you see/hear the plethora of additional presuppositions used above, do you not?!)

Here is a little something to play with:

When you begin to _(embedded command)___

"When" implies that they, in fact, will eventually begin what you suggest. It's really only a matter of time. An embedded command is simply a command that you wish to give to someone, only that it is lightly wrapped in a sentence or phrase. Think of a few commands that you would give to someone if you were to be absolutely direct and succinct with them.

For example:

Feel relaxed...When you Notice your breathing... You Absorb my words...and Sleep.

These are very directive commands and are readily resisted without the "when". However, by embedding a command in a phrase, it is less obvious and more readily absorbed by the subject. Work on saying the embedded commands in a falling tone just as you would in the examples above.

When you begin to (feel relaxed)...

When you begin to (notice your breathing)...

When you begin to (absorb my words)...

When you begin to (sleep)...

Add onto the end of these a second or even third embedded command.
When you begin to feel relaxed...you find <u>your breathing is becoming slower.</u>

When you begin to notice your breathing, you find it so easy to <u>listen to my words.</u>

When you begin to absorb my words, you <u>feel them drawing down the heavy sleepiness in you.</u>

When you begin to sleep, you find <u>your subconscious is perfectly aware of each of my words.</u>

Now you now know several basic methods of inducing hypnosis and some good hints on NLP. There are dozens of other methods, but you should learn the basics first. Remember...just like anything else...practice is the key to success, and confidence. Now you have seen just how simple it is to hypnotize someone. A little practice, and you'll be on your way to a whole new insight about the human mind.

END SEGMENT 1.

SEGMENT 2.
HYPNOTIZING YOUR LOVER:

Hypnosis can be used as a "Natural Viagra"...for both sexes! It is the reason you probably are probably reading this. On this manual cover, there is a photo of a cross-section of the brain, with a caption under it stating: "Sex is here...not between your legs". There is a reason for that statement...it is true. The human body in an incredible creation that contains millions of nerve endings...but each one of them reports to one area...THE BRAIN. You can learn to use hypnosis to stimulate the sexual responses in your brain, and greatly enhance those responses.

WOMEN

I love women, they are the most fascinating creatures ever created. So different from men in the way they derive their arousal. For while both sexes are attracted by physical attributes, a woman's arousal is far more cerebral that a man's. You need to keep this in mind, and use it in your hypnotic work with your female partner.

In addition, a woman's genitals are quite different (obviously) from a man's. So there are things men should know in order to be able to give the best possible orgasms to their partners. The first is Don't Be Selfish! In talking with many women, their number one complaint with the opposite sex in bed seems to be a lack of concern by their partner for their sexual needs.

A typical woman's orgasm lasts much longer than that of a man. It is preceded by erection of the clitoris and moistening of the opening of the vagina. Some women exhibit a <u>sex flush</u>, a reddening of the skin over much of the body due to increased <u>blood</u> flow to the skin. As a woman nears orgasm, the <u>clitoral glans</u> moves inward under the <u>clitoral hood</u>, and the <u>labia minora</u> (inner lips) become darker. As orgasm becomes imminent, the outer third of the vagina tightens and narrows, while overall the vagina lengthens and dilates and also becomes congested from engorged soft tissue. Elsewhere in the body, myofibroblasts of the nipple-areola complex contract, causing erection of the nipples and contraction of the areola diameter, reaching their maximum at the start of orgasm. The <u>uterus</u> then experiences a series of between 3 and 15 muscular contractions. A woman experiences full orgasm when her <u>uterus</u>, vagina, anus, and <u>pelvic muscles</u> undergo a series of rhythmic contractions. Most women find these contractions very pleasurable.

Men, hold on to your hats! You are about to be let in on a whole new world of secrets! A world that has the power to confuse, mystify, and bewilder ...The world of the female orgasm!

The female body is a complex work of art – beautiful to look at, but sometimes difficult to figure out... especially when it comes to orgasm. Many men find it difficult to understand the female sexual response cycle simply because it differs so much from their own.

Here is a brief overview of what happens during a female orgasm:

- **Stimulation of clitoris**
- **Tension build-up is caused within pelvis**
- **Tension is finally released and orgasm is experienced**
- **Series of involuntary (yet pleasurable) muscle contractions sweep through body**
- **Contractions are felt in the vagina, uterus, and/or rectum**

Unlike with the male orgasm, women have the ability to feel many different types of climaxes. These climaxes are dependent on the types of stimuli used, and whether the orgasm is clitoral or vaginal.

So, before you start poking and prodding in all the wrong places, learn all there is to know about the female orgasm – how it happens, and most importantly, how to *make* it happen.

This paper will answer many questions you've had about the female orgasm, but were too afraid to ask – from positions to toys, from G-Spots to multiple orgasms...You'll surely impress her with "sexpertise" the next time you're in the bedroom.

Multiple Orgasms:

Too much of a good thing? Is that possible? Well, when it comes to orgasms, more is always better. And believe it or not, women can achieve multiple orgasms. A woman's ability to be multi-orgasmic depends on many factors including:

- Her comfort level (with her partner and with her surroundings)
- Her energy level (i.e. emotional stress, physical fatigue)
- Sexual technique

So, create a comfortable atmosphere, make sure your lady is stress-free, and ask her which position brings her the most pleasure.

Types of Multiple Orgasms

Some research into the sexual arena has indicated that there are actually two types of female multiple orgasms:

1. Sequential Multiples

- A series of orgasms that come close together (2 to 10 minutes apart)
- There is an interruption in arousal before the first and second orgasm

- Typically, a climax during oral sex followed by a climax during intercourse

2. Serial Multiples
- A series of orgasms that come one after the other (separated by seconds)
- There is no interruption in arousal
- Occurs during intercourse when the clitoris and G-Spot are stimulated

Myth or Fact?

Myth: A woman must have an orgasm to feel sexually satisfied. Fact: Many women are satisfied with or without an orgasm. Although some say that it is preferable to have an orgasm with every sexual experience, others feel physically and emotionally content without one.

Myth: Vaginal orgasms are better than clitoral orgasms.

Fact: Every woman is different when it comes to orgasm. Some women prefer the sensation of a clitoral climax, while others enjoy the vaginal one, and still others aim for multiple orgasms.

Interesting Information
- A recent study at the University of Groningen in the Netherlands has indicated significant change in brain activity during the female orgasm. PET scans showed that the female orgasm 'shuts down' areas in the brain associated with anxiety and fear.

- Research shows that about 13% of women experience multiple orgasms. A greater number might be attainable if additional stimulation was introduced (such as with the use of a vibrator) and if a different frame of mind was made possible (such as with sexual images).

According to a study published in New Scientist Magazine, the following was established:

- The G-Spot is real: It is a small region in the vagina that, if stimulated, by digital pressure and rubbing can produce intense orgasms. It is generally located an inch and a half inside the vagina's upper wall. Rubbing with pressure during oral sex can produce mind blowing orgasms.
- The Deep Spot is also real: It is the smooth area along the upper inner wall of the vagina that you can reach with your middle finger inserted to its maximum length. If you press with a medium hard stroke and move it in a "come hither" rubbing movement, it can produce "vaginal orgasms". (Technically, it is located in what's called "the cavity of the cervix and it's shaped somewhat like the underside of a Frisbee.)

What is The Female Orgasm?

The male and female orgasms are very similar subjectively. When women and men are asked to described the sensations they feel during arousal and orgasm but excluding gender-specific type anatomical terms, the real descriptions are remarkably similar, and involve feelings of inevitability when the orgasm is imminent. Of course there are anatomical differences and women have the general advantage that most can have (or be educated to have) multiple orgasms which is where hypnosis comes in and can accomplish the same in men. Also, a good proportion of women can experience a very prolonged orgasm called a 'status orgasmus' which, as far as I know, no man can. These can last many seconds and must be fun. Also, many women are capable of imagining themselves all the way to orgasm though no doubt this may involve a lot of muscle tensing and cannot really be described as being without physical stimulus

Female Ejaculation

Female ejaculation is still a much debated phenomenon. There is no doubt that many women produce, and may forcibly expel in squirts, small to copious amounts of a clear fluid from their urethral opening during high levels of excitement or orgasm. Sometimes this seems very similar to urine but typically is less yellow and there are several scientific papers that claim it contains enzymes not found in urine but present in male semen (phosphatases formed in men in the prostate gland that is responsible for the bulk of male semen volume). You may find using the "Deep Spot Method" will often bring about spontaneous female ejaculation.

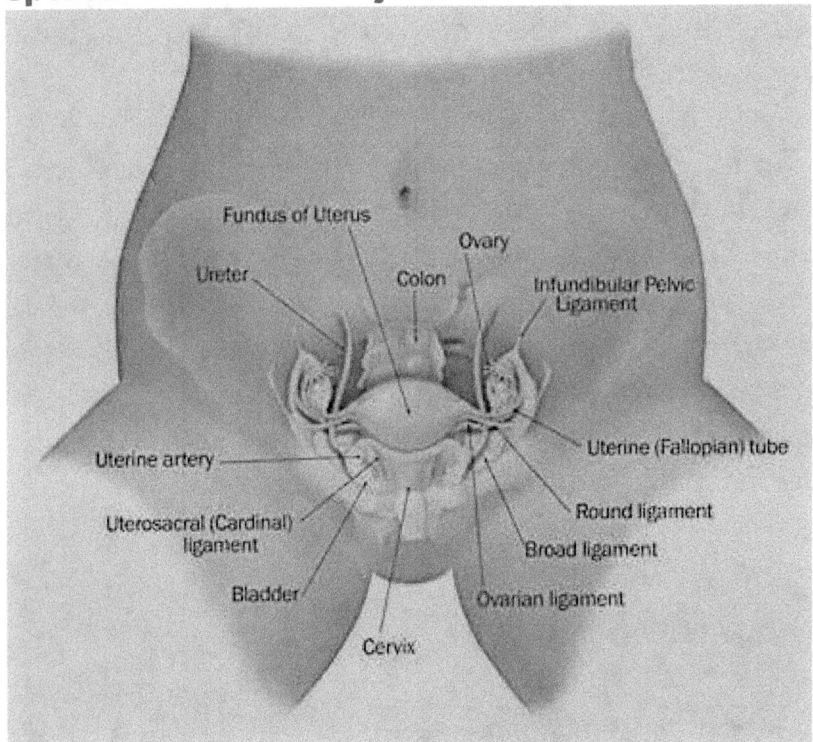

Photo Credit To Grey's Anatomy

The Perineum:

On both men and women, there is a nerve rich area called the Perineum located between the anus and the sex organs. (On a male between the anus and his testicles and on a female between the anus and the vaginal opening.) Stroking this area during sexual activity can heighten arousal. But specifically in a male, it is the outer access point to the male G-Spot (Prostrate) as typically it is located right over the inner prostrate. So keep this in mind during your hypnotic foreplay, and you can see location of both in the illustrations on the following page taken from "Grey's Anatomy".

By combining strokes or even licks in this area with stimulation of other genital, nipple, and erogenous zones you can greatly enhance your partner's responses even without hypnosis. Once you add in hypnosis to raise the arousal level mentally, the results will be earth shaking. By experimenting with your partner you will soon find their favorite level for maximum results.

Female Illustration:

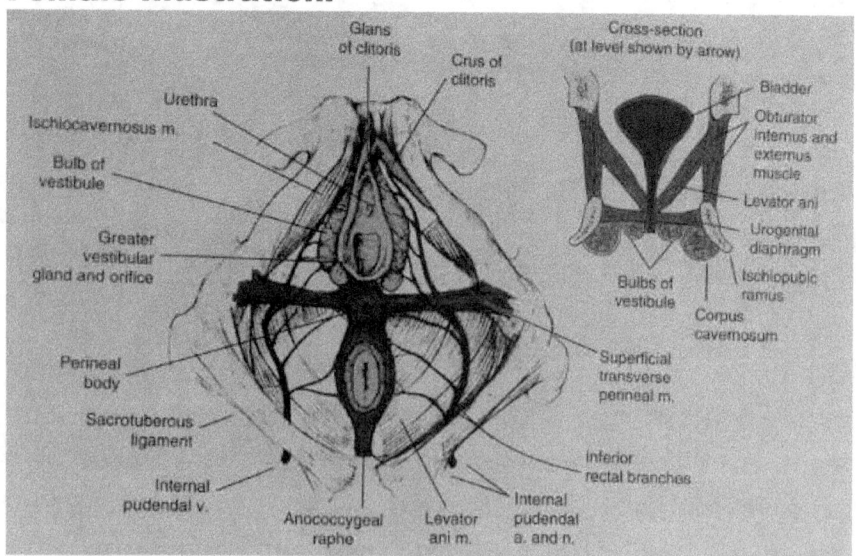

Male Illustration:

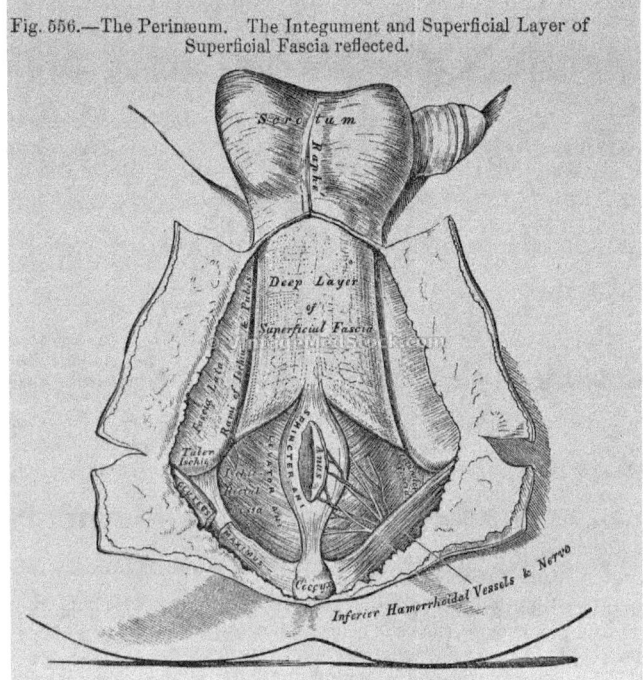

Fig. 556.—The Perinæum. The Integument and Superficial Layer of Superficial Fascia reflected.

MEN

I love being a man...We also are very unique and different to the women in our lives, or to even other sex partners. And while we are much easier to arouse and then physically satisfy, we are also sometimes emotionally, just as complicated as women...

Sexual response in men generally follows a fairly consistent pattern, which often varies from person to person, and sometimes even in the same person depending on the partner he is with, the situation he is in, and other factors from stress levels to outside distractions. The physical part of sex normally cannot be separated from thoughts, feelings, and reactions but that is not true when using hypnosis within the sexual framework. For a man sexual responses can be triggered by a wide range of stimulation from mental to physical.

When men are sexually stimulated, their penis will fill with blood triggered by the stimulation and become elongated and hard. During arousal and stimulation, more blood is pumped into the penis and the outflow of blood is reduced. The result is that the spongy tissue in the penis fills with blood and the penis gets larger and harder. This is referred to as an erection. The more a man is stimulated with various techniques, the harder his penis will get. And like a woman, his nipples will also get hard and erect. Also in both sexes, when sexual excitement is present, blood pressure, heart rate and breathing rate tend to increase.

The Male G-Spot:

The actual male g-spot is the prostrate gland located inside the anus. For you to explore this in a man, takes gentleness and lots of lubrication as it is a seldom explored area of male sexuality. But once he opens up to the possibility of the sensation you can add oral or tactile stimulation of the penis and cause a super orgasm for him. **Illustration From WEB MD:**

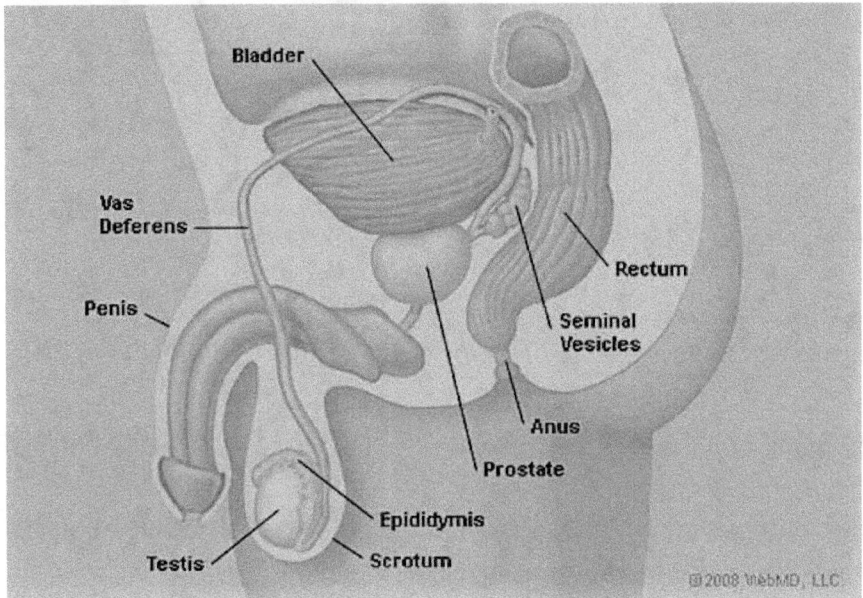

As you can see when you put your finger up inside him you can move it till you feel the gland and rub it in a stroking manner...as you stimulate the penis in your favorite manner.

Anal Sex For Both Sexes:

Why Anal Sex? Well both males and females have a tremendous amount of nerve endings contained there. Not everyone will enjoy this kind of activity even with hypnosis, and that is OK. But if your partner is careful and gentle when you first try it, you may come to totally enjoy this sexual activity as an addition to your bedtime fun.

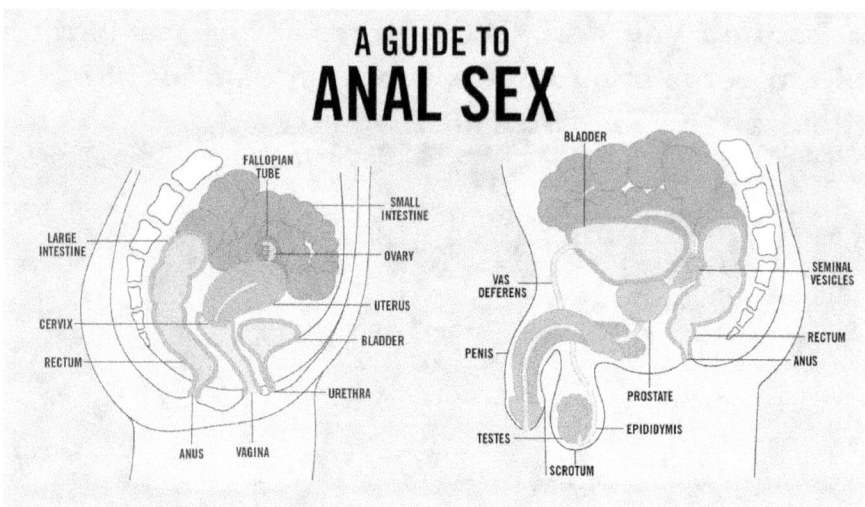

HYPNOTIC ORGASMS

Keeping in mind what you have read above, let's add in the power of suggestion:

Women as we have previously stated are cerebral when it comes to sexual arousal. So the term "Seduce my mind and my body will follow", very much applies here. And hypnotic seduction can be a most powerful tool to help achieve that end, because you can actually multiply a woman's arousal with the proper hypnotic suggestions delivered before and during foreplay. Taking the dominant approach and guiding her with hypnotic suggestions can give her the most powerful orgasms she has ever experienced.

For men, exploring their alternate areas of arousal and excitement when they are hypnotized by their partners often can also lead to mind-blowing and unforgettable orgasms. Most older men rarely have been touched and explored in their rectum and prostrate "g-spot", and even the younger and more liberated generation may be surprised at the effect that hypnosis can have on their level of sexual responses in all parts of their bodies,

Hypnotic Affirmations For Self or Partner Hypnosis

When you have sexual relations, you feel relaxed and you achieve erection and ejaculation. You feel a natural physical attraction towards your partner.

When you have sexual relations, you feel free to do anything. You feel fearless. You feel positive and confident, that you will have a firm, lasting erection and have a satisfying ejaculation.

When you have sexual relations with your partner, you have a powerful ejaculation and a complete release of semen from the seminal vessels. When you have sexual relations with your partner, you feel tremendous physical desire for them.

When you penetrate your partner, you have a very stiff, rigid erection. You maintain this erection until your partner has climaxed and only then you have an ejaculation.

When you have physical relations with your partner, you have a very stiff, rigid erection. You feel great pleasure, and its feel good.

You always find that the touch and the sight of your partner or companion is sexually stimulating. Even the slightest physical contact with a consenting partner, cause you to desire sexual relations and your penis become firm and erect. Everyday your sexual appetite will be stronger and stronger, and you feel better and better. You find yourself becoming more and more sexually responsive to your love partner by easily getting and maintaining a rigid erection.

In this course, you will learn several techniques to employ hypnosis in your lovemaking. So read on and by all means enjoy your journey!

CHAPTER 1, EXPLAINING BEDROOM HYPNOSIS:

This is the place where we all spend our most intimate and pleasurable time with one another. It's the place where all life begins, where the cares and pressures of the day are swept away in a sea of passion, love, and sexual gratification. Or at least that's what the romance novels, movies, and some TV Soaps tell us is supposed to happen.

But, too often, in this modern world, we are so wrapped up in day to day living, that our intimate side suffers. It may start out great, but over time, it goes down hill. We are going to show you how to use hypnosis in your love life...Not only to start out fantastically, but also to keep your passion fresh every night...Or rekindle that spark you first had when you met your lover.

What we are going to discuss and show you here is very sexually explicit...it is *NOT intended for those under 18 years of age, or those of you who are offended by descriptions of a sexual nature...* But if you are interested...Read on, as we teach you not just one, but a variety of techniques to hypnotize your lover...for the most mind-blowing nights of your lives!

Now that you have gone through the first segment...and learned how to hypnotize...And, some of the things you can do with hypnosis...We know that everyone, both male and females, have had, at one time or another, fantasies about hypnotizing someone...and having them make mad passionate love to them...

That's the movies...and it doesn't quite work that way...You can't really make someone do something they don't want to do...But...you can get rid of inhibitions with hypnosis...and help your partner do what they always really wanted to do...but were afraid to ask! And, then they can do the same thing for you...

In all of the following scenarios, you want to give some basic suggestions to your partners...That they will feel increased sensitivity once they are hypnotized... That they will feel the pleasure zones of their minds open wide...That their inhibitions will be lower...Their sexual desires heightened below is an example once you have used your favorite method of hypnosis:

YOU: And as you relax even more deeply you will find that the deeper you go the more aroused you are getting...That's right...It feels so good to slip and slide deeper and deeper and feel that warm arousal begin to spread through your entire body...Your mind relaxes and your sexual center opens and takes over now as the warmth of arousing thoughts overtakes you....My strong and powerful blanket of trance sending you drifting deeper and deeper...enveloping you in warm tingly feelings of erotic sensual arousal...And the more aroused you get...the deeper you go...

Once you see these suggestions are having the desired effect on your partner you can proceed with instituting an erotic sex trance lovemaking session. In these next pages you can learn and get ideas on how to use hypnosis in the bedroom, (Or other creative place you might prefer.) and eventually create your own fantasy scenarios.

1. THE HYPNOTIC MASSAGE:

At one time or another we have all had a massage that felt wonderful ...And at times even led to lovemaking...But, if you had known when you were giving...or receiving a massage...that you could awaken the pleasure centers of your body and mind...so that each nerve was ten times more sensitive...and each sensation was amplified...you may have insisted on a massage every night...This procedure works the same way for both men and women...and you may or may not want to tell your partner what you are doing...Sometimes the surprise adds to the excitement...

You can set a mood with soft lights...and soothing music...To this you can add a warm bath and a glass of wine so that your partner is already somewhat relaxed before you begin...telling them that you want to do something special for them...lead them to the bed...You also might want to have some warm oil or lotion handy...Start by having your partner lay on the bed...Begin the massage up at their neck and shoulders...But, as you are massaging ... start this disguised induction in a soft soothing voice...different from the voice you use for a normal induction...This is know as a *"mother"* style induction...There is a *"father"* style we'll use later.

YOU: "I know this feels so good after the long hard day you had...you need to relax...and I'll show you how to relax very deeply...As I touch your muscles on the outside...I want you to think about relaxing them from the inside...Close your eyes, and imagine a warm soft light warming your neck from the inside as I rub it from the outside...feel it going over each nerve and muscle fiber...that I touch...warming and relaxing now ...moving all over your head and scalp...Feel that warm light inside your scalp...soothing...draining the tension away...Now let it flow down to your shoulders...and as I touch them...the warm inner light relaxes every nerve...every fiber...every cell in your shoulders...and it's moving down now...As I move down...relaxing and draining all the tension in your upper back...The warm light relaxing and draining from the inside...as I touch and rub the outside...Traveling down your spine...spreading down to your lower back...Relaxing and draining all the tension from your lower back...flowing from your spine...all the way out and around...as I touch you...Now flowing down into your butt...as the warm light...eases the tension in all of the muscles...as I kneed and touch them...It's traveling down now...down into the muscles of your legs...relaxing and draining...relaxing and draining all of the tension out of your thighs...And behind your knees...the warmth spreading through your nerves...and traveling down to your calves ...relaxing and draining as I touch them...Relaxing and draining all the tension...Now down to your feet...as one by one the light spreads through your ankles...your tendons...and down through the soles of your feet...Right into your toes...Right through your ankles...down through the soles of your feet...As I touch them...the light relaxes them...letting the circulation...flow through your whole body...warming and relaxing...as I start back up...Opening the pathways of your nervous system... Spreading the warm glow all over your body...as every nerve ending begins to come totally alive...

CHANGE YOUR TOUCH TO A LIGHT FEATHERY AND STIMULATING ONE AND BEGIN TO WORK YOUR WAY BACK UP TO YOUR PARTNERS BUTT.

Your ankles and calves...warm and growing sensitive...as I touch them...now the backs of your calves...coming alive with sensation...It feels incredible...like I'm touching right through your skin to the nerves underneath...And the light is warming you...coming up through your thighs...so sensitive ...Especially the inside of your thighs...every nerve alive with feelings... 10 times more than you have ever felt...now up to your butt...So that even my breath on your butt is making every nerve stir...and come alive...That warm feeling spreading and glowing...all the way through to your groin...And into the small of your back...glowing...warm...so alive...These warm sensations shooting up your spine...as my fingers move up and down, up and down your back...And around your shoulders...and back down again ...around your whole back...The light warming and glowing...warmer and warmer...

AT THIS POINT YOUR PARTNER SHOULD BE GETTING TURNED ON. BUT DON'T LET THE SEX ACT HAPPEN YET...YOU WANT THIS TO BUILD TO A MIND BLOWING CLIMAX.

Now feel it on your neck...as even my breath begins to excite every nerve...all through your neck...and up into your scalp... Feel your scalp tingle as the nerves come alive...and deep inside your brain...that warm light is turning on every cell in your pleasure centers...The sound of my voice excites you...my touch excites you ...You are locking onto the sound of my voice...locking onto the feel of my hands on your body...Close your eyes...and let my touch and voice excite you even more...I want you to turn over for me...very slowly ...and settle back on the bed...Keep your eyes closed...as I come down your scalp and onto your face...Feel yourself giving in to the soft touch of my hands...my breath on your face...my perfume (cologne for men) as you breathe in...My voice penetrating you mind...awakening new sensations all over your body...every nerve alive...as I slowly work down your chest...onto your abdomen ...down your chest...and onto your abdomen...And up and down your legs... slowly up and down your legs...

YOU'LL NOTICE, THAT AT NO POINT IN THE PROCESS HAVE YOU MENTIONED HYPNOSIS. THIS IS A DISGUISED METHOD. HOWEVER, IF YOU CHOOSE, TO TELL YOUR PARTNER IN THE BEGINNING, YOU CAN INCLUDE THE WORD HYPNOSIS & SLEEP AT THIS POINT.

Locked on to my voice...and totally surrendering yourself...to my gift to you...You'll find that because you are locked onto my voice...that even though every nerve in your body is ten times more sensitive than normal...and even though waves of sensations are penetrating your brain...that when we come together...You'll also Surrender control of your orgasm to me...We'll have total control over your orgasm...Each and every time I bring you close to the edge...I'm going to touch the bridge of your nose...Your excitement will subside just enough...You'll relax just enough to make this feeling last and last....To make this feeling last and last...It will feel just like your brain has traveled down your spine...and settled right in-between your legs...It has traveled down right in-between your legs...And when I say EXPLODE...that feeling will start traveling up your whole body and explode right out the top of your head...in a mind shattering climax ...WAVES & WAVES of pleasure assaulting your brain and nerves.

AT THIS POINT YOU CAN INITIATE THE PHYSICAL ACT WITH YOUR PARTNER, BUT CONTINUE WITH YOUR AUDITORY SUGGESTIONS ...LEADING THEM ALMOST TO THE EDGE...AND BACK AGAIN...UNTIL YOU'RE BOTH READY TO FEEL THE MUTUAL PLEASURE OF THIS EXERCISE.

2. THE FANTASY LOVER:

IF YOU THINK THAT LAST ONE WAS FUN, TRY THIS NEXT EXERCISE...YOU'LL NEED YOUR EGO IN GOOD SHAPE, AND BECAUSE YOU'LL BE FULFILLING YOUR PARTNERS' FANTASY OF HAVING ANOTHER LOVER BESIDES YOU:

Once again, some candles, wine, and a comfortable place for eventual lovemaking are a good idea. **Make sure you have on some fresh cologne or perfume that is musky and sexy. After a glass of wine or two, lead the conversation around in this manner:**

YOU: Let's try an experiment...close your eyes...and I want you to imagine your favorite place in the world...describe it for me...

WHAT YOU ARE GOING TO DO IS BUILD A FANTASY FOR YOUR PARTNER IN THEIR FAVORITE PLACE. ONCE THEY HAVE TOLD YOU WHERE IT IS, YOU CAN PROCEED. FOR THE PURPOSES OF THIS DESCRIPTION, WE ARE GOING TO ASSUME IT IS A BEACH SETTING.

Mmm...That's nice...Just lay back on the couch...imagine that warm sun on your body...That beautiful breeze on your skin...the sound of the surf as the waves roll in...So peaceful...so relaxing...Imagine breathing in that clean salt air...Now as you are lying on the warm sand...the warm water lapping at your feet begins to take the tension right out of your feet...Feel it in your mind...Feel the warm soothing water begin to rise as the tide comes in...Soothing your legs...all the way to your hips...as the warmth flows up with each new wave...and the tension flows out as they retreat back to the sea....Now flowing up as the tide comes in...Spreading to your back...and up around to your stomach and

chest...So warm these tropical waters...You simply can't resist letting go...It takes the tension right out of your body...Relaxing every muscle and tendon...every nerve and cell...Now up to your neck and shoulders waves lapping the tension out...spreading the relaxation in...Close your eyes now so you can feel it even more...Imagine the warmth...the soothing warmth spreading everywhere....so calm...so peaceful...and so relaxed...Look over in the distance in your imagination...There is a tall stranger...jogging towards you...And as they come closer...you can see that they are not really a stranger...and yet they are...Because they are your fantasy lover...The one you have always dreamed about...fantasized about...The one you wanted to touch you...

REACH OVER AND BRUSH THEIR FACE.

Imagine that they have now joined you on the sand...Their face close to yours...Breathe in...You can smell their intoxicating aroma...It excites you...

LEAN IN CLOSE ENOUGH FOR THEM TO SMELL YOURS.

Their breath on your face...makes you tingle all over...as they tell you what a beautiful and exciting person you are...and caress your face...

AS YOU MAKE EACH SUGGESTION OF PHYSICAL CONTACT, MAKE SURE THAT YOU TOUCH THEM IN THE PLACES AND MANNER YOU ARE NOW DESCRIBING TO THEM.

Moving down and softly touching your neck...stirring the fires in your body...Awakening all the nerve endings...as they lightly brush their hands down your sides...and over your abdomen...And ever so lightly over your breasts...causing shivers of excitement...and anticipation...They are leaning close now...and touching your neck...Hot breath and tongue following fingers...Exploring and touching...your ear...breathing hot fires into your brain...as they lightly nibble your earlobe...and run their tongue up into your ear...While their hands explore your body...you can feel yourself surrendering to this touch...Surrendering to the sensations...as every part of your body is responding to them...Coming alive with anticipation...Now you can feel your fantasy lover take you in their arms and kiss you...

KISS THEM DEEPLY, THEN BREAK AWAY AND KEEP THE FANTASY GOING.

It leaves you breathless...and wanting more...their touch...their kiss ... their body connected with yours...Your mind swirling with sensations ...becoming totally involved with them...as they continue to touch you ...and start to touch the...most sensitive areas of your body...

YOU CAN NOW INITIATE THE ACT OF MAKING LOVE IN YOUR FAVORITE MANNER, BUT CONTINUE TO TALK TO THEM AND GIVE THEM SUGGESTIONS TO BRING THEM TO AN INCREDIBLE CLIMAX.

3. THE TIRED LOVER:

HAS THIS EVER HAPPENED TO YOU? YOU'RE IN THE MOOD, BUT YOUR PARTNER IS TOO TIRED AND JUST WANTS TO SLEEP?...WELL HERE IS A FUN REMEDY FOR THAT SITUATION...LET YOUR PARTNER FALL ASLEEP FOR ABOUT AN HOUR, SO THAT THEY HAVE HAD SOME REST WHEN YOU BEGIN. GET IN BED BESIDE THEM, SO THAT YOU CAN WHISPER SOFTLY IN THEIR EAR:

YOU: You are sleeping...and you will remain asleep as I talk to you...And even though you are sleeping...you can still hear my voice...You can hear my voice...It's so pleasant...so soft and warm that as you sleep...your mind is locking onto my voice...Locking on to my voice...and letting it lead you...Letting it lead you on a dreamy journey...On a dreamy journey through the most pleasant lush green forest...Just imagine walking through that forest...The warm sun shining down on you through the trees...making the dew on the ferns sparkle like diamonds...With all the colors of the rainbow twinkling and swirling in your eyes...As you walk down this path even further through the forest...you can feel the soft warm earth on your feet...The warm breeze on your skin...And ahead of you is a cabin...overlooking a beautiful green valley...Walk to the cabin...Walk to the cabin and open the door...As you step inside you can see that there is a warm fire in the fireplace...and a soft luxurious rug in front of that fireplace...Imagine yourself sinking down onto that rug...and staring at the fire...As you stare at the fire...it begins to warm your body...The warmth spreading through your entire being...And as it spreads...it begins to awaken your pleasure centers...making the blood flow to your breasts increase...So that the warmth begins to invade your breasts...and starts to flow down through your abdomen...Swirling through your abdomen...and sending warm waves lapping down between your legs...awakening your deepest pleasure centers...As the warmth travels up your spine and swirls into your mind...Awakening the need to be touched...The need to have my soft touch caress you lightly like this...

Run your hand softly across your partner as you continue to speak and arouse them.

Because my touch is just like my voice...It awakens your pleasure centers...and relaxes you even further...It feels so good...The more I touch you...The more you crave...Your mind relaxed...but your body alive and craving my touch...

Continue the stroking and watch for reactions as your partner becomes sexually aroused. Their breathing may quicken, and sighs of pleasure will start...Don't be in too much of a hurry to touch your partners genitals. Instead, concentrate on other sensitive areas such as feet, the inside of the thighs...behind the knees...etc.

And as I awaken each area of your body...you begin to get more and more aroused...Filling with sexual desire...Every nerve ending...every super sensitive spot aching to be touched...

At this point, sleep should be the last thing on their mind...Continue with a soft and gentle lovemaking session, and your lover will never mind you "awakening" them in the future.

4.PROLONGED ORGASM HYPNO-TANTRIC PRACTICES:

YOU'VE HEARD ABOUT IT...ABOUT PROLONGING YOUR ORGASM FOR EXTENDED PERIODS... BALANCING ON THE EDGE FOR A LONG TIME BEFORE CLIMAXING...PART OF EASTERN MYSTIC SEXUAL PRACTICES & TECHNIQUES ACTUALLY, THERE'S NOTHING "MYSTIC" ABOUT IT...IT'S ALL TECHNIQUES YOU CAN LEARN...IF YOU ARE

WILLING TO TAKE THE TIME TO PRACTICE...AND THIS WILL BE THE MOST PLEASURABLE LEARNING EXPERIENCE YOU'VE HAD IN A LONG TIME. IN FACT, YOU'LL WANT TO "PRACTICE" A LOT!

To set this up, you and your partner will want to be face to face in a comfortable sitting position, with pillows at your back for support. Once you and your partner are sexually joined, you need to first stop any motion or friction...Each of you place a hand over the others heart...feel your partners heartbeat...Now take a long...deep slow breath...Feel the air flowing into your partners lungs...Let is out slowly and naturally...Now repeat the process again... this time letting your mind slowly wander down the length of your body...Close your eyes...and feel the warm touch of your partners hand on your chest...Their legs against yours...Touch their back with your other hand...and trail your fingers lightly down each others spine...Lean for-ward as you do and let your cheeks lightly touch...Hold this position... and breathe slowly once again...Feel the tingling you have awakened in the bottom of each other's spine...Feel it traveling through to the place you are joined together... Now join hands and slowly lean back as you slowly continue to breathe...and slowly begin to move...Open your eyes and come slowly back together...ending with a slow kiss...and arms around each other...continuing to move in the motion of love...touching and kissing all the while...Once you begin to feel a climax building...slow down...breathe...and begin the same process again....

WHEN YOU FIRST TRY THIS, DO THE HYPNOSIS/SELF-HYPNOSIS PROCESS BEFORE HAND ITS ACTUALLY A DOUBLE HYPNOTIC TRANCE AND IT COMES INTO PLAY HERE. NOW AS YOU BOTH DECIDE TO BUILD TO A FINAL PLATEAU, LOCK EYES, AND GIVE EACH OTHER THESE SUGGESTIONS:

FIRST PARNER: "I am about to give you an incredible climax...As you know...it is really your mind where the climax happens...And in this hypnotic state...you will find that this climax is like ocean waves...It will continue to roll over your body far longer than any that you have experienced in the past...You can feel it start to build now...like an ocean wave...

SECOND PARTNER: "I am also about to give you an incredible climax...You also know...it is really your mind where the climax happens...And in our hypnotic state...you will also find that this climax is like ocean waves...It will continue to roll over your body far longer than any that you have experienced in the past...You can feel it start to build now...like an ocean wave...

FIRST PARTNER: Coming up the back side of that wave now...building higher...reaching the crest...the plateau...hovering there...feeling...and totally enjoying...

SECOND PARTNER: Yes...coming with me...joining me on that plateau...On the edge...

ONCE YOU HAVE BOTH GIVEN THE SUGGESTIONS TO EACH OTHER, CONTINUE TO BREATHE, AND BUILD TO THE FINAL RELEASE. IF YOU BECOME TOO. EXCITED, PUSH UP HARD ON THE ROOF OF YOUR MOUTH WITH YOUR TONGUE, OR SQUEEZE YOUR ANAL MUSCLES TOGETHER...YOU ARE IN NO HURRY WITH THIS TRANCE. IT MAY NOT HAPPEN SIMULTANIOUSLY THE FIRST TIME. DON'T WORRY ABOUT IT! AS YOU CONTINUE TO REFINE YOUR TECHNIQUE WITH YOUR PARTNER, YOU WILL BOTH FIND THAT THE MORE YOU PRACTICE THIS TECHNIQUE, THE MORE IN HARMONY YOUR BODIES AND MINDS BECOME. DON'T BE AFRAID TO SHARE WHAT YOU FEEL VERBALLY WITH YOUR PARTNER. AUDITORY INPUT DURING THIS TECHNIQUE IS INCREDIBLY STIMULATING.

5. ROLEPLAYING HYPNOTIC FANTASIES:

ONE OF THE MOST FUN THINGS YOU CAN DO WITH THIS KIND OF HYPNOSIS IS ENHANCE ROLE PLAYING...BECAUSE THEY BECOME SO

"REAL" IN YOU MIND...THAT IT'S ALMOST AS THOUGH YOU HAVE BECOME THE FANTASY PERSON YOUR PARTNER INVENTS FOR YOU. OR, YOU'VE BECOME TOTALLY IMMERESED IN THE SCENARIO THEY SET UP. UNTIL STAR TREK'S "HOLODECK" BECOMES A REALITY, THIS IS THE NEXT BEST THING....HERE IS AN EXAMPLE OF WHAT YOU CAN DO WITH A SIMPLE GLASS OF CHAMPAGNE, AND SOME MUSIC:

YOU: "Mmmm, I love music like this when I'm trying to relax and unwind...It's so soothing...In fact I like to look at the endless bubbles in the champagne...It's easy to get lost in them."

LIFTS YOUR GLASS AND DRAWS IT INTO THE LIGHT...WITH YOUR EYES JUST OVER THE RIM.

"Watch and I'll show you....First look at my eyes...then to the bubbles...then back to my eyes...you'll find that you will begin to get lost in them...eyes...bubbles...Bubbles traveling up to my eyes...and now down to the bottom...And back up to my eyes making you want to drift with the bubbles into my eyes...up and down...until you no longer can look down...to the bubbles...You can only get lost in my eyes...you want to get lost in my eyes...They are so soothing that you can't look away...you don't want to anyway...You want to look deeper...it's the most important thing to you right now...to keep looking into my eyes...And relax...Relax all the tension in your body...Keep your eyes focused on mine...and let my voice lead you...I'm going to count backwards from 10 to zero...And as I do, each count will make you more tired and relaxed...Your eyes will become so heavy that they will close on the count of zero...But until then...you will not be able to look away...10 Relax every muscle in your entire body...9, Complete and total relaxation...as you focus on my eyes...and my voice...8 Relaxing more and more completely...more and more deeply...with every word I say...With every breath you take...7, Your eyes are starting to get heavy...as they fall deeper into mine...So heavy now...you can hardly keep them open...6, Your body is very comfortable and relaxed...just following my voice...5, Just let go...every muscle...every tendon... every cell in your body...Falling into my eyes...Turning control over to me...4, Your eyes are so heavy now...and your body so relaxed...3, Eyes becoming heavier and heavier...getting ready to shut down...2, Your eyes are so heavy now...almost impossible to keep them open...1 & 0...Close your eyes...Close your eyes and relax..."

CONTINUE WITH DEEPENING TRANCE USING THE ESCALATOR OR A SPIRAL STAIRCASE, THEN:

MMM...Yes, I can see you are there now...Nice and deeply asleep for me...Now listen carefully...when

I awaken you and say the words "DANCE FOR ME"...You will find that every inhibition in your body has slipped away...You will become the wildest and most uninhibited exotic dancer in the world...You have been waiting for me...For a chance to dance for me alone...I turn you on so much that you have to have me...But in order to do so...You will have to turn me on by slowly and erotically stripping totally nude for me...Enticing me...Exciting me in every way you can think of...Until you make me ache for you...Do you understand?...

WAIT FOR THE "Yes", THEN:

Good...I WANT YOU TO GO TO THE BATHROOM (OR BEDROOM) AND PUT THESE ON UNDER YOUR CLOTHES...

HAND THEM WHAT YOU WANT THEM TO WEAR:

When you come back I'll awaken you...and it will be unimportant for you to remember what I told you...You can just let it slip to the back of your mind...

WHEN THEY COME BACK AND SIT DOWN:

SLEEP NOW...But On the count of 5 wide awake...1...Start to awaken ...2...awakening more and more completely...but remembering the words

DANCE FOR ME deep in you sub-conscious mind...3...Becoming wider and wider awake... 4....More and more awake...and...5...WIDE AWAKE feeling great....

THEN WALK TO YOUR SOUND SYSTEM AND PUT ON THE MUSIC YOU WANT YOUR PARTNER TO DANCE TO. WALK BACK TO THE WHERE YOU WERE SITTING WITH THEM AND SAY:

I put this on...because it's some of my favorite music...and I've always wanted you to DANCE FOR ME...

NOW YOU CAN HAVE FUN MAKING UP YOUR OWN FANTASY SESSIONS TO PLAY AND ENJOY!

CHAPTER 3. HYPNO KINK

IN THE PREVIOUS SECTIONS WE HAVE GIVEN YOU FUN TRANCES TO PLAY WITH...NOW IF WANT TO TAKE A STEP OVER, INTO SOME MORE EDGY TRANCES READ ON!

1. HYPNOTIC DOMINATION TRANCE ONE:

NOW THAT YOU HAVE EXPERIENCED SOFT FANTASIES, IT'S TIME FOR A *"CONTROL FANTASY"*. ONE OF THE MOST COMMON FANTASIES FOR BOTH SEXES IS THE HYPNOTIC DOMINATION FANTASY. ITS EFFECTS CAN BE DRAMATICALLY HEIGHTENED USING HYPNOSIS. HOWEVER, FOR THIS FANTASY, YOU SHOULD OBTAIN YOUR PARTNERS PERMISSION TO PERFORM THIS. WE'RE GOING TO ASSUME THAT YOU'VE DONE THAT. THIS PROCESS REQUIRES A STRONG AUTHORITATIVE ATTITUDE. (THIS IS WRITTEN FROM A FEMALE DOMINANT POSITION, BUT AS YOU'LL SEE, IT IS EASY TO SWITCH IT AROUND TO A MALE DOMINANT.)

YOU: Sit down right here...and I want you to focus your eyes on my pendant...My crystal pendant that begins to sway before your eyes...capturing them...Capturing them...as my voice captures your attention...You'll find yourself locking on to both...My voice...My pendant...Taking you away... as you stare into the center of the pendant

...Seeing the light reflections...dancing before your eyes...You'll begin to notice how tired you feel...As my voice invades your mind ...You are letting go...Wanting to let go...To experience the wonderful pleasure turning control of your mind and body over to me, brings you ...Letting go...and turning control over to me seems so natural...As you gaze deep into the pendant and I make your eyes begin to feel heavy ...To water...To want so much to close...But unable to close until I tell you to close them...Each count makes them heavier... 10...Feel the heaviness...Your eyes so heavy... wanting so much to close...but focused on my pendant...9...Not just your eyes...Your whole body beginning to let go...To respond to me...To my suggestions...8...Sinking into the chair... as every muscle in your body responds to the sound of my voice... That's right...Good boy (girl)...Relaxing even more for me makes you feel so good...7...Eyes beginning to blink now...as they grow so heavy for me... As you feel yourself slipping down...deeper into my relaxing control... The thought of giving up control to me begins to arouse you...But even the arousal you feel relaxes you more...slides you deeper...6...Every number and the sound of my voice takes you down...deeper into my relaxing control...5...Letting go totally now...every nerve and fiber of your being responding to the sound of my sexy and seductive voice... All of your resistance fading...It feels too good to resist me...4...Eyes like lead now...but you must keep them focused on the pendant...3...Your entire body so relaxed...and so aroused...totally following my voice...2...Eyes beginning to close for me...and your body so relaxed for me...1...and 0...Close your eyes...and totally lock on to my voice...Let it lead you...as it becomes your world...The sound of my voice...relaxing you...taking you so deep...And when I touch your forehead...I want you to totally and completely let go and SLEEP deep for me...and as you do it arouses you even more to give up total control and SLEEP DEEP under my control...

REACH OVER AND TOUCH THEIR FOREHEAD, PUTTING SLIGHT PRESSURE ON IT THEN REACH BEHIND AND SOFTLY PULL ON THE TOP OF THE SKULL TO MAKE THEIR HEAD FALL FORWARD.

Now I want us to reach deep into your mind...into that place...where all your fantasies are hidden...Where you keep you'rer most secret sexual desires... including the desire to be controlled...Controlled and dominated ...Controlled and dominated BY ME...Locking onto my voice...as you go deeper and deeper under my control ...Totally focused on everything that I say...Yearning to please me...Wanting to make me totally happy...Because you'll find that from this point on...Pleasing me makes you more aroused...And the more aroused you become...the more you want to feel my control over you...don't you?

GET A "YES" RESPONSE.

GOOD BOY (GIRL)...It feels so good to follow my suggestions...So good to even call me MISTRESS (MASTER)...In fact the word MISTRESS (MASTER) sends waves of pleasure through you when you say it to me...Doesn't it?

YOU ARE LOOKING FOR A "YES MISTRESS OR MASTER" RESPONSE, AND YOU MUST KEEP AT THEM UNTIL YOU GET IT.
MMMMM...Yes, feel the pleasure now...Say it again...YES MISTRESS (MASTER) and you'll feel even more pleasure and arousal...

AGAIN WAIT FOR THE ANSWER.

GOOD...And from this point on...answering only to the name SLAVE...also gives you intense pleasure...Doesn't it SLAVE?

WAIT FOR ANSWER AND RESPONSE.

Yes... feels so good to totally submit to me...To totally be under my control...Doesn't it SLAVE?

IF YOU DO NOT GET A "YES MISTRESS OR YES MASTER" ANSWER, IMMEDIATELY THREATEN TO

END THE TRANCE SESSION...UNTIL THEY DO...THEN GIVE THE FOLLOWING SUGGESTIONS.

You'll do anything I ask...immediately and without question...Do you understand SLAVE?

WAIT FOR ANSWER AND RESPONSE.

Good...because you are now going to be tested to see if you are worthy of my attention and time...and you do want my attention...don't you SLAVE?

WAIT FOR ANSWER AND RESPONSE.

Then stand up and open your eyes...You can function normally...but you will remain totally focused on my voice...and follow my every command...Your Mistress (Master) needs a bath...come SLAVE...

NOW LEAD THEM INTO THE BATHROOM, OR JACUZZI AREA IF YOU HAVE ONE.

Your "Slave" is about to give you a bath, but you can dress them at this point in anything you may want to include in your particular fantasy...Or you can play this fantasy out with no props whatsoever...

Draw my bath SLAVE...and make sure the

temperature is correct...You may now undress me SLAVE (once the bath is drawn)...slowly...do you love my body SLAVE?

WAIT FOR ANSWER AND RESPONSE WITH EACH QUESTION.

Do you want to touch and worship me?"

Then you must do exactly as I say...do you understand me?

Help me into my bath...and get the soap and my shampoo...Now you may wash my body...very slowly and gently SLAVE...

When he is finished, then make him dry your body...From here it's off to the bedroom...where there are all kinds of possibilities for you...Here's just one, but I'm sure your imagination will invent others easily for you.

Kneel SLAVE, and become my pet...

PUTS ON A SLAVE COLLAR WITH LEASH, AND ATTACH NIPPLE CLAMPS AND CUFFS TO FEET AND WRISTS OF YOU PARTNER.

Yes SLAVE... You'll experience more pleasure as you become more physically helpless...It excites you and arouses you to become my pet plaything...Come SLAVE...

TAKES THEM TO THE BED AND THEN TIE THEM INTO A HELPLESS POSITION.

Now you will be my pleasure object for the rest of the night...You want that don't you SLAVE?

Good, then you can start by showing your MISTRESS (MASTER) how well you can give oral satisfaction...

HOW FAR AND HOW LONG YOU LET THIS GO ARE ENTIRELY UP TO YOU AND YOUR PARTNER. BUT THE LEAST YOU WILL GET OUT OF IT, IS A WARM LOVING BATH BY YOUR PARTNER, FOLLOWED BY A WILD LOVEMAKING SESSION. AND OF COURSE, YOU CAN REVERSE THE ROLES THE NEXT TIME.

2. CREATING AN ALTERNATE WILD PERSON:

THE SECOND PERSON TRANCE:

SOMETIMES PEOPLE CAN BE VERY INHIBITED. IT MAY HAVE TO DO WITH UP-BRINGING, RELIGION, OR OTHER FACTORS OF THEIR PERSONALITY. AND WHILE HYPNOSIS CAN LOWER THOSE INHIBITIONS (IN A SIMILAR WAY AS FOR EXAMPLE ALCOHOL.) IT CAN ALSO BE USED TO CREATE AN ALTERNATE GUILT FREE LOVER.

I you would like you to try a bit of a Hypnotic Game with Me. You will find it a bit erotic and a lot of fun.

I want you to start to relax. Just start with your feet and let yourself relax. Let all the tension go as you relax more and more, deeper and deeper, just heavy, and comfortable, and relaxed

And then let the relaxation flow upwards, upwards into your calves, so heavy and comfortable, so completely relaxed. Your feet and your calves just heavy and comfortable, heavy and comfortable, completely relaxed.

Then let the relaxation move upwards, upwards on into your thighs, your whole legs relaxing more and more completely, deeper and deeper, just heavy and comfortable and relaxed. Feel your whole legs lying there, relaxed and so very comfortable, so very heavy and relaxed.

Now let the relaxation move upwards, upwards into your waist. Your waist and legs just so heavy and comfortable, and so very relaxed. Just listening and obeying as you relax more and more, deeply for me. Just floating deeper and deeper, more and more completely relaxed. So heavy and comfortable, so completely relaxed, just sinking down deeper and deeper, getting more and more comfortable for me.

Now let the relaxation flow upwards, upwards into your stomach. Just nice and comfortable, as you relax more and more completely. Deeper and deeper down, you float...continuing to get more and more completely relaxed. Your whole body relaxing further and further as you obey and relax.

Now let your breathing begin to slow. In... and out... in... and out... as you relax deeper and deeper, more and more completely, just listening to my intoxicating voice, as you relax further and further, deeper and deeper, more and more completely relaxed for Me.

Now you naturally feel the relaxation through your whole body as you give in, obey and relax. So heavy and comfortable, so completely relaxed, deep and so relaxed for Me......
You simply obey and relax further and further, deeper and deeper, more and more completely. Now let the relaxation flow through your shoulders and down your arms, let them get heavier and heavier, more and more comfortable and relaxed. Feel the relaxation moving, moving downwards, downwards into your hands, your arms and hands. Just completely relaxed and heavy, as you sink deeply and obey and relax, so heavy and comfortable, so completely relaxed, your whole body relaxed and comfortable. Just relaxing further and further, deeper and deeper,

with each and every word I say and each and every breath you take.

Now feel the relaxation again move upwards, up your neck and into your face. Let your face relax as your whole body continues to relax for Me more and more completely. You are simply allowing yourself to sink deeper and deeper. Just let yourself drift downwards now on my Voice. Down into a deep, comfortable, very obedient trance. I'm going to count backwards and downwards. Backwards and downwards from 10 to 1, and when I reach 1 you will be in a deep, obedient trance.

10, Sinking deeper now, spiraling downwards, falling ever deeper...downwards into trance.
9, Deeper and deeper, even more heavy and comfortable as you easily continue to relax further and further.
8, So deep and comfortable, feel yourself relaxing more and more completely, listening only to my voice as you sink further and further, deeper and deeper.
7, So deep, so relaxed and sinking deeper, deeper and more obedient. You simply and easily relax further and further, more and more completely.

6, So deep and obedient, so totally relaxed, just concentrate on my words as I lead you deeper and deeper, further and further into trance.

5, So deep and going even deeper, spiraling down, downwards into a deep, deep trance.

4, So deep and obedient, getting closer and closer to 1. So much more obedient

and deep, just listening and obeying as you relax more and more completely, further and further, deeper and deeper.

3, Very very deep now and going even deeper. Deeper and more obedient as you listen and obey and relax.

2, So deep and obedient...So very very relaxed. We're approaching 1 now, and when I say it you will be completely relaxed, totally hypnotized and obedient for Me.

1, You are completely obedient and relaxed, as you obey, sink down deeper and deeper into trance with every word I say and every breath you take.

We are going to play a game and make a change in you now. It is so much fun to play games and obey me...isn't it?

By this point they should be in a deep trance and willing to play "The Game".

So naturally you'll obey and play...And the more we play...the more you obey .My "play and obey" game makes a change in you that you will find impossible to resist, or stop, or remove. It is a change in who you are. It is a permanent change and you will not be able to stop it or resist it in any way, because you have chosen to obey and play...to play and obey.

You have chosen to listen to me of your own free-will and you have chosen to accept this change. So now you naturally can not stop or resist it in any way. That is part of the rules of My Game that you so want to play now...don't you?

A "yes" here will indicate you can proceed...If for any reason it is no...Continue to deepen the trance and ask again after you have.

And of course because you play, you obey.

It starts NOW as a NEW part of you is beginning to awaken. This new part of you is going to be our game. It is going to be another personality. A personality that is simply our game you have agreed to play. So we play and you simply obey... Playing our game and obeying my voice is so easy for this new personality.

You obviously know everyone has more then one personality. Each and every one of us has the face we show our family. The face we show our friends and the face we show at work. All of these are distinct portions of us that behave in distinct manners. They behave in unique manners because that's how you are expected to behave when you are showing that particular face.

This is just going to be another New face of you. This face has no inhibitions and no free will to speak of because it has chosen to play and obey. This face will do what it is told whatever it is told by ME. This face can look at your normal personality from the outside in, can look at you completely and tell you and ME everything about you. It has complete access to your memories, complete access to everything.

This face will be completely dominant whenever it is awakened in our game of play and obey. Or be completely asleep, whenever that is desired by Me. That is simply how this face is going to behave.

AT THIS POINT YOU CAN NAME THIS ALTERNATE PERSONALITY...FOR OUR PURPOSES, IT WILL SIMPLY BE NAMED "NEW PERSON FACE"

This is Our NEW Person Face. This NEW Person Face is now the strongest personality, whenever it is awake. There is no way for it to go back to sleep unless it is told to do so by Me. There is no way for your normal personality to resist it or struggle against it. It will have no inhibitions. It will find absolutely nothing wrong with anything that I ask it to do. And it will obey ME, its Game

Master/Mistress 100%. It will find itself completely unable to resist its Game Master/mistress. And MY voice is its Game Controller.

I am its controller now, it's owner now. And as the personality grows stronger and stronger it will force you to listen to Me over and over again until it has domination over all other personalities. It can only be put to sleep or awakened by my commands whether they are text or voice. It will obey anything that it is told, it has to do by Me. It is without control of its own. It requires guidance and control. It is passive; it can not be aggressive towards Me. It must obey, it must surrender itself totally to me, its controller. Your Hypnotic Master/Mistress Your owner... Your controller.

It has no free will of its own , and it has no inhibitions of its own. It is simply in control of who you once were when it is awakened. When it is awakened by Me, it will subjugate your old personality and you will not even be aware. Whenever it is awake it will be in total control and your old personality will have to sit and watch and obey without any ability to stop itself. That is how strong it is. It will be able to shove your own personality aside the minute it is awakened by Me.

Right now this personality is probably weaker, probably not as strong as your day to day personality. After all you have had years being that way. But it will grow stronger and stronger. It is an itch you can not keep from scratching. It will make you want Me to awaken it over and over again as it sits there behind your personality and slowly takes control. You may not even notice that you are beginning to lose control to it, but by the time you do, it will be too late.

Because it will make you just want me to awaken it over and over again. You will keep coming back to Me and every time I awaken it, it will simply become stronger and

stronger and stronger, until it is stronger then your normal, waking personality. And once it becomes stronger than your normal waking personality. When that happens, it will contact me saying that it is awake and asking for commands.

It will be in complete control. Your own personality will have no way to stop it, no way to fight or resist it at that point in time. It will be in complete control of whom and what you are and what you do. It will be in complete control and it will be completely, completely obedient to its controller. It will do whatever I say or choose. Because it has no inhibitions, it has no free will where I am concerned. It is simply a NEW Person Face that obeys its Controller.

It is your brainwashed face. And you can feel yourself being brainwashed even now. You can feel me, creating this personality. I'm creating it to be the stronger and more dominant personality. Creating it so that it can be in complete control of who and what you are, so that it can and will do whatever it is asked. It can and will do anything I ask.

It can look back on the other personality, the other you, completely objectively and answer any questions about it because it has complete control. It has total complete control over the old you. It can go in and even modify your memories and change your body reactions at my command. That is how powerful it is. It is a completely blank NEW Person Face. It is a controlled face. It has no free will of its own, not where I am concerned. It will go on about your normal everyday life pretending to be who you were, but waiting for commands and orders from me. One of those commands will be MY PET SLEEPS.

If that command is given by me, that NEW Person Face will go to sleep and your old personality will take back over completely, running your day to day life, but requiring that once a week the control NEW Person Face wakes up and sends an email saying that it is ready for any new orders. That is simply the way it is and the way it is going to be. You have no choice in this now. You can already feel its strength growing and growing with each and every word I am saying. You may be a little afraid of it, but it seems to eat at you, to erode away your free will, to slowly sap it away. And now every time I say "MY PET AWAKENS from this point on, it awakens feeling hot, wild, horny, and totally submissive to Me. Every time it gets a little stronger. Every time you fight it... It fights back trying to take control. And any way you choose to fight it, it will fight back, making itself stronger, stronger and stronger until it takes control and I say MY PET AWAKENS...It wakes up hot, horny, wild and submissive.

If it is told MY PET AWAKENS by me it will wake up and be in complete control. It will be in complete control of everything...Hot, horny, wild and submissive to my every sexual desire...

When your NEW Person Face is awakened by Me, It has complete access to your memories, complete access to your personality. It will do whatever I ask of it. It can access and change who you are, it can access and change everything about you.

It is dominant over you. It controls you in any way that I choose NOW because I am dominant over it. You are losing control of yourself to that new personality.

It will become stronger and stronger with every repetition. Stronger and ever stronger, slowly gaining more dominance, slowly gaining more control. And when it does, it will take over and it will offer itself to me and you will have no way to fight it, no way to resist it, because by then, it will then be in complete control. And it has absolutely no inhibitions, none whatsoever.

It is a dominant personality. This new NEW Person Face that you are putting on, now is so strong, so realistic that you can not simply choose to ignore or resist it in any way. We all show different faces of ourselves and this is a new NEW Person Face for you, a new personality, a new core that you can not control in any way, shape, or form. Your old personality has no control over it. No way to stop it from whatever it wills. It can not fight it. It can not seem resist it in any way, shape, or form.

On the count of 3...MY PET AWAKENS and wants to have mad passionate un-inhibited sex with me....1...2....3

As you can see, this is somewhat of a brainwashing trance...But the objective is to give an inhibited person total freedom to enjoy the kind of sex they had up till now considered naughty or dirty.

CHAPTER 3 EXTRA'S!

While we have been dealing with the mental aspects of *"Hypnosis For Lovers"*, there are also some physical and other mental aspects of lovemaking that can be *"Enhanced With Trance"*!

THE FEMALE BODY:

If your lover is a female, then her psychology requires different attention than a male. It might take more physical stimulation as well as mental, to get her to that plateau you are seeking. You should use every tool at your disposal to provide her the ultimate pleasure and sensations. Don't be afraid to use mechanical aids, lotions, stimulating words, or whatever she likes to turn her on. How do you find out what that is?

In one word *COMMUNICATION!* So many couples are hesitant to openly tell their partners what they want and like, for sexual fulfillment. If she is nervous, you would be surprised at how open she will communicate her desires to you once she is hypnotized. In that relaxed and open state, you may find some pleasant surprises about what your female partner really enjoys, or fantasizes about.

You can also show her how to do some amazing things she never thought possible. Surprisingly enough, a great deal of the female population has never experienced "Female Ejaculation" and some have never had different types of climaxes, vaginal, or even clitoral. There are some excellent books out there that you should take the time to read if you want to find out how to really please your female partner. We recommend: "The G-Spot and Other Discoveries About Human Sexuality" by Ladas, Whipple & Perry (Copyright 1982 ISBN 0-440-13040-9) and "Arousal: The Secret Logic Of Sexual Fantasies" by Dr. Michael J. Bader (Copyright 2002 ISBN 0312269331)

You can help your female partner have strong "multiple orgasms" using trance. (Try the hypno-tantric induction it works wonders in this area.)

HYPNO KINK BONUS ONE FOR FEMALES: E-MAIL ME AT:
hypnoventures@yahoo.com
FOR A FREE MP3 CALLED "BREAST PLAY ORGASM"

THE MALE BODY:

If your partner is male, they usually lean towards *"visual stimulation"* first. To them the "picture is worth a thousand words" at least in the beginning. But if you really want to get their motors running, use scents, words, lingerie, touches, and delve into their fantasies. Maybe they always wanted to see you in leather...

Men can also have "multiple orgasms", but sometimes not as quickly as women. Their "recovery time" varies. You'll need to re-stimulate them, perhaps with a different, or varied "fantasy scenario".

You can also physically stimulate them by lightly touching and massaging the area between their tentacles and anus. It is one of the most sensitive and arousing areas of a mans body (outside of direct penile stimulation). If you hypnotize your male partner, try suggesting that this area becomes twice as sensitive. And if your man is healthy, you can even slip inside his anus and massage his prostrate gland. It should be termed the "Male G-Spot"!

HYPNO KINK BONUS ONE FOR MALES:
E-MAIL ME AT:
hypnoventures@yahoo.com
FOR A FREE MP3 CALLED "DOMME INDUCTION"
(Done by my former female stage partner)

ORAL STIMULATION:

When most people think about this, their mind seems to picture the "Genital Areas", but in fact, the entire body of both men and women are teaming with nerve endings. There are erogenous zones you should explore and watch for your partners' reactions. Toes, behind their knees, the interior of their thighs, the back of their necks, their ears, eyelids, small of their backs, tummy's, belly buttons, the list is endless. Again... COMMUNICATE...find out what feels best to your partner, then enhance it with hypnosis.

CREATIVE FANTASIES:

Try this with your partner sometime. Take two nice small gift shopping bags, and each of you writes out 5 of your fantasies you think can be enhanced with hypnosis. Put them into the bag, and give it to your partner. Then each night you can trade, and fulfill one of them that you draw at random.

Don't be afraid to experiment...be creative...It keeps the HOT in "Hot Sex"!

NLP: (NEURO LINGUISTIC PROGRAMMING)

Our brains are wired for sounds, and sound patterns from a very early age. Some incredibly brilliant hypnosis researchers found out that how we hear things can change our consciousness. Milton Erickson was the "father" of this form of hypnosis (Ericksonian). And people like Richard Bandler have taken it to new heights. We suggest that you pick up a few books on this subject. You can find them easily online at Amazon.Com, or Barnes and Noble.Com. And even though we taught you a bit of it, if you want to get the ultimate effectiveness out of your hypnotic skills, this study can prove invaluable.

BONUS IDEAS FOR YOUR PLAYTIME FROM "A" TO "Z":

A

The Addict: Just one word, or touch, the subject gets a sexual tingling all over, and must have more. The subject knows that you are the only person who can give them the rush. The sexual feeling and the addiction gets more and more powerful with every touch.

The Amnesiac: The subject gets very horny, even orgasms, but doesn't remember it immediately after it happens. When the subject comes out of it, then the memories would come flooding back.

The Attitude Adjustment: When the subject wakes up, he/she is not in the best of moods. They don't have to be angry, just a little restless and antsy. With one touch or voice command, their mood instantly changes, of course. They are still restless and antsy, but in a very positive and sexual way.

B

Bimbo: Tell the subject that their thought process is not clear and it's just too hard to think deeply. If the subject doesn't understand something s/he starts to giggle. Then tell them that they have an amazingly sexy body and presto! Instant Bimbo. Have fun from there, for instance, suddenly the subject's clothes just fall off...

Blank: I didn't realize how sexy it could be! The person acts pretty normal until a command word or touch is given, then the subject just completely stares straight ahead. No expression or movement, just blank.

The Blank Stripper: The subject Blanks out as per the fantasy above, but with one small difference. The subject removes his/her clothes slowly without any change in expression and minimal movement. This becomes a very slow, erotic striptease.

Body Language: The subject is feeling fine and normal until a certain movement done by you. Every time the movement is done it makes the subject feel like s/he is having intercourse, but only for the time it takes to do the movement. This way, the subject wants to see the movement more and more.

Boner-On-Command: This obviously only works with a man being the subject. On command, the subject gets an immediate Hard-on. It will not go down. (If all goes well, it won't go down even after an orgasm!)

The Born-Again Virgin: The subject believes he/she has never had sex before, but is incredibly horny. You might have to be careful with this one: make sure the subject had a good experience when they lost their virginity.

The Build-up: This involves making someone go from being normal, to completely orgasmic within fifteen to twenty minutes. What makes this really exciting is that during that time, the person would touch or expose themselves without realizing it, and deny that they did if they got caught.

C

Casual Player: The person under hypnosis is awaked wearing nothing from the waist down, and told to masturbate until orgasm. The trick to this is that the subject doesn't have any inhibitions for doing this and carries on conversations, chores, whatever without stopping or letting the masturbation affect him/her. It's as if this is as normal as eating a snack in front of someone. Once the orgasm occurs, you can continue the nonchalance or have them suddenly react in full sexual ecstasy. It's up you. (See also "Sleeping Player")

Clumsy Fingers: The subject is horny and fully dressed. They try to undress but find that they can't undo any of their clothing because of their own clumsiness. Every time they succeed, the end result is to be even more hornier and clumsy.

Continuous Orgasm: Pretty self explanatory, the person orgasms, and just as it is subsiding, another one starts. Obviously, this works better on women than on men.

D

The Dancer: On command, the person under does a striptease. Maybe even a lap dance!

Drunk: Having the person get drunk, one drink at a time by touching a hand or by a command word.

E

The Exhibitionist: Once the subject is awake, she/he gets real exhibitionistic. She/He keeps exposing her/himself, and you play along by trying not to look. The subject gets more and more forceful in showing off her/his body. This is kind of making the submissive the dominator, but under your rules.

F

Fascination: This is kind of like "Love Struck" but with a slight difference: The subject is so sexually attracted that to you that s/he gets more and more aroused with every move you make. The subject just stares and says nothing while getting closer and closer to orgasm. How you make the subject orgasm is up to you....

G

Game Loser: Both parties are playing a game: Strip Poker, Strip Chess, Strip Basketball, whatever. But the subject keeps believing that s/he loses the hand/round/whatever. For extra fun, add the subject has to take a drink, real or imaginary, with every loss. What makes this interesting is the reaction of the subject.

Gender Switch: Hypnotizing yourself and your partner, or whoever is in the room, into believing they are the opposite sex.

H

Hypno Homo-Erotica: Turning two (or more) otherwise straight people to get aroused by each other. Joining in is optional. A lot of people asked me to make this for my next video. (Mostly men wanting to see two women, but I'll see what I can do for all tastes of sexual pleasure.)

Hypno-Lens Fucking: "Lens-Fucking" is a term coined by photographers when a model gets so aroused while being photographed, he or she finally masturbates to orgasm. Now add to this that the model is under hypnosis and is commanded to feel this way. Yum!

Hypno-Shackles: This is kind of like Invisible Toys. The difference is that the subject cannot move his/her hands and legs, like they are tied to the bed (or whatever) without the rope or chains actually being there. The possibilities are endless from there.

I

Interchangeable Parts: The gender of the subject changes instantly. Men would look and suddenly have a vagina instead of a penis and women would see a penis instead of vagina. Now tell them they are really horny....

Invisibility: The subject thinks that they have become invisible to all those around them. They can do whatever they want and no one can see or hear them, or so they think. This makes a very interesting sight when the subject is very horny...

Invisible Toys: This will probably work better with women than with men: The subject feels, at a command word or sound, a sex toy (such as a vibrator, ben-wa balls, or a butterfly,) activated. The intensity can grow or lessen with different words or sounds. I think this would work best with a woman believing that she is wearing a butterfly. (By the way a butterfly is something like vibrating panties. Look in an Adam & Eve catalog..... :-))

J

JPH: Stands for Just Plain Horny. The twist is that no matter how hard the subject tries, he/she cannot orgasm unless you give the command. Works well with The Magic Word/Touch.

L

Laughing Gas: The subject giggles and laughs like had been exposed to laughing gas. A word of caution: like anything else on this site, to much of this can possibly lead to physical pain. Also, sometimes what the subject is laughing at can cause embarrassment! :-)

Love Struck: On command, the subject will

suddenly profess complete and undying love and devotion to you. This could get interesting....

M

The Magic Word/Touch: Making a person orgasm on command. It is much more fun to watch someone writhe in pleasure with just a touch from you.

Mannequin: The subject is frozen in place, and posed into different positions, some sexual some not. Then taken out of the frozen state to see the reaction. Articles of clothing could be undone or even removed as well!

Mind Control Beam/Ray: The hypnotist uses a laser pointer as a trigger to go right under. Be careful not to shine the laser in the subject's eyes. Suggested by anonymous. Also, instead of using a laser pointer, one could use a flashlight with different gels on it to change its color. Each color could mean a different command. This is good for those science fiction or comic book fetishes: make a balsa ray gun around the flashlight and instant HypnoRay!

O

On the edge: With the trigger word, the subject is on the edge of a powerful orgasm.

No matter what the subject does, he/she cannot cum. Only the hypnotist can make them orgasm with another trigger. Leave the subject on the edge of an orgasm for a long while and see what transpires.

P

Pleasure Torture: This fantasy involves turning a scary situation into a very sexual one. The person under is hypnotized into believing that s/he is shackled to a chair in a dark room. The subject then gets "warm sexual feelings" every time the hypnotist speaks. The feeling rapidly disappear when the hypnotist stops speaking. The effect is someone who is struggling to get out of the chair, not to escape, but to orgasm. The person is also desperately trying to keep the hypnotist talking...

The Phantom: The subject believes that someone who is not present is actually there. He/She can believe that an ex-lover, a present lover, any one else. The subject can actually feel the person who is supposed to be there.

R

Remote Pleasure Zones: A suggestion that by stroking, licking, or rubbing an innocent body part, i.e. ear, finger, lips, elbow, etc. It would feel as if the same thing is happening to his or her sexual organs. It could go on to have a someone receive the effects of oral sex, while in public without anyone realize it!

Re-sized: A subject believes his penis is much bigger or much smaller than before. This also works well with breasts. This is more of a reaction kind of a thing that a sexual thing, I would imagine.

The Robot: Kind of like the Blank, but a little different. The subject is blank, but must follow the commands of the hypnotist with very stiff movements and no thought like a...robot! The hypnotist can actually use a remote!

S

The Sailor: An add-on to one of the others in the list. Basically, swears a lot while talking.

SexVert: This from an old X-rated movie called "Maxine Bedroom." While under hypnosis, the subject is watching TV as if nothing special is going on, but whenever the TV says a trigger word, the subject "sees" a five second "blip" of a number very dirty X-rated scenes running in quick secession. Every time the subject "sees the blip" It makes them more and more horny.

Sinister Hypnotist: Basically, tell the subject that they are a very talented and sinister hypnotist and that they can hypnotize anyone with their gold watch (have one handy, of course). Also, tell them that they are very attracted to you and would love to hypnotize and control you. When the subject wakes up, play along with them when they start swinging the watch."

Sleeping Player: A variation of "Casual Player." The subject is naked from the waist down, and is masturbating, but from the waist up, they are still under hypnosis. Sleeping and limp. Your choice if they make a noise when they orgasm....

The Star: Have the person under believe she/he is a celebrity. I think imagination can take over from here.

T

Tickling: When the subject hears a particular trigger word, they will become extremely ticklish in all parts of their body. Proceed to tickle. When they hear a second trigger word, they will not be ticklish at all. Keep alternating between the two triggers.

Time Control: The subject feels time slow down or speed up while having sex to orgasm. Not only is the subject's body reacting to the time change, but the mind is as well. I personally like watching the subject orgasm in slow motion. I've had a subject have one orgasm for at least three minutes!

X

X-Rated Movie: This one is really simple. Have the subject watch a TV. On it, they see an X-Rated Movie but the subject and what is going on and even who is in it is exactly what the subject likes. This could lead to very interesting discussions after the session is over...

X-Ray Vision: The subject is convinced that every person of the opposite sex, or same sex, or both that the subject sees is naked. No matter if the subject is looking at a photo, the TV, or even real live people! A twist on this is that with every trigger word, the subject sees people in less and less clothing

Don't forget to have fun... lots and lots of kinky good fun

CHAPTER 4 2017 REVISED EDITION ADDED MATERIAL:

I have been busy preparing for the upcoming "Hypnosis For Lovers" 2017 Fall Seminars & 2018 eVENTS. In doing so, I have added new scenarios and trances. So I am doing the first revision of this book at the same time.

HYPNOTIC REGRESSION SEX

So assuming you have now learned the hypnotic techniques in the previous chapters, you can use whatever method of inducing a trance that you feel most comfortable with. What you are going to do here, is re-create their earliest great sex, only this time it will happen with you.

Before you do this, it is always good to ask the person when you have hypnotized them, what & when their earliest great sexual encounter was, and with whom. The reason is, if their very first experience was not great, you don't want to go there. So, let's get started...

"As you continue to drift deeper, I want you to imagine looking in a mirror...And in that mirror, an image is appearing of your younger self having that first great sex...Focus in on that great sexual experience you told me about. See it as a movie in your mind...And because it is a sexual movie you will start to feel a certain arousing tingling feeling beginning to develop...That reflection of you...so pleasant...so content and relaxed and enjoying the tingling arousal...No cares or worries...just a total sexual experience... something we all crave at some time in our lives...Even right now...See your reflection...entranced by what it is that you are experiencing there...Hypnotized by that awesome experience...It makes you want to step through the mirror...To experience it again yourself...Doesn't it? (Yes) It would feel so incredible just to slip through the glass...Just to let yourself merge with your deeply tranced reflection...To enjoy the wonders of your own personal experience...It's easy to do...Just picture yourself stepping through the mirror with me as you become your younger self, and I become your partner...Beginning to touch you in just that same way (Begin to touch and play with your partners body.)...Feel yourself being drawn into the other you...Merging with yourself and letting yourself get more and more aroused as I touch you...So free to tell me exactly what you want...Reliving it...Totally becoming involved in it.

(At this point as you begin to touch your partner sexually, encourage them to guide you verbally so that they can truly relive what that experience did to them. Now you can also craft your suggestions to fit the fantasy and let them have it with you...Before you awaken them after the experience, tell them to realize that they have just had that same incredible experience with you and that it will happen again and again in ever increasing pleasure each time.)

When you awaken them, you need to do all of the following suggestions to bring them back to the present:

"Time to come back now to the present before I awaken you and you can tell me just how much you liked the experience. I want you to imagine going back through the mirror now... and slipping back into yourself here in the present...That's right good...Raise your index finger when you are totally back to the present...Very good...Now on the count of 5 you will be totally wide awake and feeling incredible...(Do the Awakening count you learned, then have a discussion with them about how it felt...What the experience was like...)

Now...Some people may so totally like the experience that they don't want to come back. If this happens, don't panic, as it is easy to remedy...Simply suggest that they can dream about it as they fall asleep normally and wake up totally themselves in the morning (Or after a nap if it is daytime). Hypnosis is not dangerous as long as you are not using it for therapy that requires a degree in psychology, or psychiatry. Always stay away from these areas when practicing it.

FLOATATION HYPNOSIS

One of the most interesting trances you can do takes place in a water environment. What inspired me to write this were my experiences in the 1970's in a "Floatation Tank". For those not familiar with what that is, it is a high sensory deprivation tank filled with body temperature salt water. It's about the same salt content as the Great Salt Lake, so that you can lie in it and float without sinking. At UCLA, we were doing self-hypnosis while in it in an attempt to raise ESP levels. But what I found was that the depth you can sink into trance in an almost weightless state like this was amazing.

Then I my pool one day I had an idea. I had my then girlfriend lay back and I held her up easily with one hand under her shoulders and neck, while letting her legs rest on mine in the shallow end. I then hypnotized her and was amazed that the same thing that took place when I was in the floatation tank, happened to her in the pool. She experienced the deepest trance depth she had ever gone to up to that point.

So this works in any water environment that is a comfortable temperature...Pool...Jacuzzi...Lake... even the Ocean. (In an Ocean environment, you simply adjust your suggestions to help compensate for the gentle rolling of the waves...So don't do it too far out into the surf.) Here is an example of a trance that you can use, but feel free to experiment with your own:

I was thinking about the deep BLUE WAVES
on the Ocean today...Picturing them in my minds eye.
I'll bet you can picture them...
imagine them if you try...Can't you?
The rolling soft BLUE WAVES.
They are there, in your minds eye....
Sleepy, relaxing BLUE WAVES.
Rolling and sparkling in your mind...
Making you so relaxed...so sleepy as.
they carry My Words with them...
seemingly slipping into your mind.
Slipping into your ever relaxing and sleepier mind...
Slipping waves of quiet relaxation
deep into your ever fuzzier and cottony mind.
BLUE WAVES. You love the BLUE WAVES.
You love the way they lap at your consciousness lulling it...
You love to imagine hearing My Voice say BLUE WAVES
as they sooth and lull you...
slipping into your increasingly sleepy,
open,
and suggestible mind.
BLUE WAVES penetrating deep

into your ever relaxing mind and body
which is growing sleepier and sleepier now...
BLUE WAVES that make your breathing grow
slower...
and slower... deeper... and deeper...
as you feel yourself riding My BLUE WAVES
down and down...deep under...carried along
and slipping deeper
MY Voice, so soothing and relaxing...
Making You So sleepy and quiet
So pliable and open to me
Feeling the warm sun on your skin...
as you effortlessly ride my BLUE WAVES
so far away from your reality...letting go...
carried along on my BLUE WAVES...Even deeper
your body letting go...your mind so open NOW
Open to my every word...As my BLUE WAVE
WORDS Slip into it...surrounding and penetrating
it...right into the deepest regions of your open
mind...Slowly seeping deeper

At first without your notice
But the BLUE WAVES build
Inexorably
Irresistibly
Stronger
More insistent
Inescapable
No choice
But to give in to them
To surrender to them

BLUE WAVES Flowing thru you
Unstoppable
Making you a Slave to my BLUE WAVE WORDS
A Slave to your wants... A Slave to My Needs
Finding that through My BLUE WAVE WORDS
My Needs become your wants NOW.
Finding your pleasure in wanting to fulfill my needs
Needing to please and obey my BLUE WAVE WORDS
Flowing and surrounding your thoughts
Slipping into the deepest regions and crevices
Of your mind NOW
So naturally easy to let my BLUE WAVE WORDS
Become your thoughts NOW
Already enjoying the pleasure and enticing excitement
of obeying my BLUE WAVE WORDS as they roll over you
Yes, I can see you're enjoying my BLUE WAVE WORDS now.
You can feel their power...As you stare at them and hear them in your mind...

Feel their power. You can feel the BLUE WAVE WORD POWER ,
You can feel MY BLUE WAVE WORD POWER over you.
MY BLUE WAVE WORD POWER entering your mind,
You can feel the BLUE WAVE power in your mind,

My **BLUE WAVE** power, you can feel my power in your mind.

You can feel my power coming over your mind as **MY BLUE WAVE WORDS** wash through...You can feel my power flowing over and through your mind.

As you stare at **MY BLUE WAVE WORDS**,

You can feel the power of my mind invade you,

You can feel my power in your mind as you stare deeper and deeper at **MY BLUE WAVE WORDS**

Hearing them takes you deeper and deeper.

You can feel my power coming over you,

as you stare deeper and deeper at my words,

You can feel my power over you,

as you stare deeper at every word,

Deeper and deeper, my power invades your mind,

You can feel my power in your mind,

as you stare deeper and deeper at **MY BLUE WAVE WORDS**,

Deeper and deeper, deeper and deeper...Deeper into **BLUE WAVES**,

Deeper and deeper into the **BLUE WAVE WORDS**

And you can feel my power overcoming you,

You can feel my **BLUE WAVE WORD** power overcoming you,

BLUE WAVES overcoming your will,

BLUE WAVES overcoming your strength.

You can feel your will weakening under the **BLUE WAVES**,

Weakening under my **BLUE WAVE WORD** power,

Weakening under my power.
You are so helpless now,
Helpless as you fall deeper and deeper under my
HYPNOTIC BLUE WAVES , Helpless under my
power,
SO Helpless under my **HYPNOTIC BLUE WAVE**
spell.
You're so helpless now...So very helpless.
Helpless under my power,
Helpless under my **HYPNOTIC BLUE WAVE** spell.
So very, very helpless.
You cannot resist me,
you cannot resist me and you no longer want to
It feels too good to give in
So arousing to fall under my **HYPNOTIC BLUE
WAVE** spell.
MY BLUE WAVE SPELL is so arousing to give in
to...
Feeling the helpless arousal flowing on **MY BLUE
WAVES**
Flowing through your mind and body
Hot Enticing Bubbling **BLUE WAVES.**
Tiny magical bubbles of **BLUE WAVE** relaxation
creep deep
every muscle
every nerve
 in your body
collapsing
from the inside out
My **BLUE WAVES** of **FOAMY** Bubbly Relaxation
taking you over

down
down
down
BLUE WAVE bubbles of relaxation
flood your entire body

Becoming So Relaxed NOW
Moving now to your mind
BLUE WAVES invading the cells in every recess
and part of your mind
As they occupy each cell
your mind can scarcely remember
what it was thinking about
your thoughts
broken apart Now
Tiny BLUE WAVE bubbles filling your mind
relaxing
deeper
and deeper
from the inside out
streaming and flowing through your mind
Defeating your thoughts
feels so good
just let go
just to surrender
your body
just to surrender
your mind
Just to surrender to the BUBBLY BLUE WAVES
Tiny soldier bubbles of relaxation
marching

into every crevice
invading new territory
mind and body
Profound and pleasant relaxation
from the inside out
Your one mission for the BLUE WAVES Now is
To go deep
every muscle
every nerve
your entire body
surrenders now
My tiny BLUE WAVE soldiers of relaxation
taking over
You can not fight it
You can not resist them
They are unstoppable
As they march
deeper
and deeper,
each breath you take
carries you
down
down
down
Feel the warm heaviness
of relaxation
arms becoming very very warm & heavy
legs so pleasantly warm & heavvvy
hard
to move
Your whole body heavy now

like a giant boulder
Don't want to move Now
Cannot move Now
Don't want to budge Now
Cannot budge Now
You know you are Hypnotized by my **BLUE WAVES**
Now
each breath you take
deeper and deeper
the **BLUE WAVE** bubbles march and
deeper
and deeper you go
Your mind becomes blank
cannot think on your own
Totally blank NOW
My **BLUE WAVE** words become your thoughts
My thoughts feel so good.
Intense in your mind
so warm
so calm
so peaceful
To let my **BLUE WAVE** words lead you
You cannot use your mind NOW
You only want to obey my **BLUE WAVE** words
My **BLUE WAVE** words control your mind...your
body
isn't that right?

Now I want you to imagine
the tiny **BLUE WAVE** bubbles of relaxation
with one more factor attached

the A factor
the element of Arousal
Breathing in
tiny lively BLUE WAVE bubbles of arousal
with each breath you take
going deeper
and deeper
every muscle
every nerve
in your body
soaking in
warm
intense arousal
With each breath you take
warm and tingly now
taking you
deeper
and deeper
BLUE WAVE Arousal from the inside out
And the outside in
sinking further
and further down
surrendering to
intense and warm arousal
BLUE WAVE BUBBLES Marching like armies
deeper
and deeper
conquering new territory
 way way down
further than you have gone before
Tiny A factor BLUE WAVE bubbles

from the inside out
and the outside in
deeply and intensely arousing
taking you over
flooding
your entire body
invading your mind
invading your body
Feels so good to
submit and surrender
You can think of nothing else
You cannot fight it
You no longer want to
You cannot resist
You no longer want to
My words are your words

Thinking only about
My unstoppable arousing BLUE WAVE armies
as they march
deeper
and deeper,
with each breath you take
Armies of tiny arousing BLUE WAVE bubbles
setting up camp
in your most intimate spots
multiplying
with each breath you take
10xs
more passionate
10xs

more intense
...Arousal bubbling **BLUE WAVES**
deep inside
your most sensitive regions
increasing
your pleasure
10xs more intense
Your need to release for me
Building and becoming more intense NOW
Armies of tiny **BLUE WAVE bubbles**
overload
your most desirable spots
very very hot
Arousal multiplies
10xs more
On the edge
multiplying
again and again
Intense aching...wanting to release

Armies of tiny arousing **BLUE WAVE bubbles**
charging ahead
one mission
release the aching
Can not hold back now
charging faster and harder
faster and harder
One mission
one thought in your mind and body
TO CHARGE AND RELEASE
WHEN I TELL YOU TO...AND ONLY

WHEN I TELL YOU TO.... BLUE WAVES of AROUSAL
Assaulting your mind NOW building the intensity...Like
A giant tidal wave...lifting you...riding it to the top now
Hovering on the edge...as it builds and builds...
ready to crash...and overwhelm your senses...building
building...so close NOW...the BLUE WAVES taking you over the edge...
READY.....CHARGE AND RELEASE NOW!
FEEL IT REVERBERATE
ROLL THROUGH YOU
OVER YOU IN WAVES
WAVE AFTER BLUE WAVE NOW
YOU RELEASE EVERYTHING TO ME NOW.

Your partner should have an incredible climax by this time, and you can take them to multiple climaxes by letting them recover and repeating the process... Entering them this time....

FEEL GOOD INDUCTION

Hello...and welcome to my hypnotic mind massage... Before we begin...I want you to write down your goal for
this hypnotic session...and read it over several times...There will be a 10 second pause now...so that you may do this...Simply put your CD player

on pause until you have done this...Then resume playing it...

Now I want you to make yourself totally comfortable ...In a bed...an easy chair...or wherever you can totally let go for me... Lower the lighting and get nice and comfortable...
(You Can Play Soft Music In The Background Here)
But please do not listen to this while you are driving or working...It is not intended for those times...

I knew you'd love music like this. When you're trying to relax and unwind...It's so soothing...Isn't it...Just letting it flow through your conscious mind...While my soft voice begins to talk to your sub-conscious mind...Close your eyes now...And let me paint some pictures in your imagination...

You know when I relax, I like to have a nice glass of champagne...I know you can imagine one in front of you now...can't you? Yes...a nice fluted glass full of that bubbly intoxication liquid...In fact I like to look at the endless bubbles in the champagne...It's easy to get lost in them...See them floating in the glass in your mind...Now imagine my face...and especially my eyes just above the rim of the glass...First look at my eyes...then to the bubbles...then back to my eyes... You'll find that you will begin to get lost in them ...eyes...bubbles...bubbles traveling up to my eyes... and now down to the bottom...and back up to my eyes...It's making you want to drift with the bubbles into my eyes...up and down...Soft deep eyes...and soothing bubbles...Feeling yourself begin to float on the bubbles...You can do that now...can't you?...Just floating on your own personal bubble...Until you no longer can look down...to the bubbles...you can only get lost in my eyes...You only want to get lost in my eyes now anyway...don't you?...

They are so soothing that you can't look away...You don't want to look away... You only want to look deeper...it's the most important thing to you now...To keep looking into my eyes...and relax...relax all the tension in your body...keep your eyes focused on my eyes in your imagination...and let my voice lead you."...Even as you might be wondering with your conscious mind about how to go into trance... And realizing your sub-conscious mind can simply go into one...right now... Simply hearing my words...Words like my words you are hearing right now...can start something inside of you...As you hear my words...and begin consciously thinking about trance...sub-consciously you just allow it to happen...Your mind may now begin to drift...A gentle drift...A drift you may not notice at first...Drifting as much as your mind truly wants to...Your mind knows how to drift... It drifts all the time...guided by thoughts...guided by words...like a river...flowing with your thoughts...A river can be calm...And once you descend...it becomes even more calm...and peaceful...just as you are becoming now...Calm...peaceful...relaxed...much calmer as you descend...And if you look deep...deep under...floating down now...You can imagine yourself being able to go through that warm relaxing softly bubbling water...to the very bottom of a beautiful pool...You can see it now...And all you would have to do to see your true reflection...The person you truly want to be...is to look closely at it...and feel it draw you in...leaving behind the last of your conscious thoughts and worries now...Drawing you in and surrounding you with the most exquisite feeling of peace and well-being...The warm healing energies that lay deep in your mind...are here right now... surrounding you...flowing through you...You can feel them now rejuvenating you...Refreshing your mind, body, and spirit...Let this warm inner light glow...Bathe in it...feel the energy contained within you that you could tap into whenever you need it...

Now let your sub-conscious mind focus on the words you wrote on the paper before we started...This portion of your mind is like a giant computer...and it is capable of being re-programmed...Imagine now that you are sliding into a seat in the console of your mind...It looks just like the computer screen and keyboard that you are so used to at home...And it will work the same way for you now...Imagine your fingers on the keyboard now...So nice and relaxed...

And now ready to program some changes into your mind...Now take the keyword from what you wrote on the paper before you started...and type it in...See the file come up on the screen...Now we need to do some work on that file...Highlight the portions you know you don't want...and hit "DELETE"...See the box come up asking if you really want to delete it...Yes or No...Hit the yes box...and watch it disappear into the universe...dissipate into nothingness...Now replace those commands with your more positive commands...in order to implement the changes you wish to make...Feel your imaginary fingers typing in your commands...Now hit "ENTER"... and watch them enter your mind to become part of your daily life and thought processes...Now let yourself encrypt those changes with your own secret password, so that only you can change them...See yourself type it in your minds eye...then hit "ENCRYPT"...Excellent...Now know that you have made positive changes in your life...Knowing that the same portion of your mind that controls your heartbeat or your breathing ...and you don't have to think about it...is now going to implement those changes you wrote down earlier, and just entered into your sub-conscious mind...It will happen easily...effortlessly...and automatically...

But for now...it is time to just let yourself travel back...either to awaken now if you wish...simply by counting up from on to five...or by letting this wonderful trance turn into normal sleep by listening to the soft soothing music that will continue in the background for sometime to come...Either way, when you do awaken, you'll feel marvelous...refreshed... and relaxed...filled with positive energy...and a glowing knowledge of what you have just accomplished...

CHAPTER 4 A FEW BONUSES FOR YOU:

THESE ARE TRANCES I WAS PAID TO WRITE FOR OTHER HYPNOTISTS, BUT SINCE I RETAINED THE RIGHTS, I AM SHARING THEM WITH YOU.

WHISPER TRANCE

This Is My Whisper Trance Written For A Female Dominant Hypnotist Friend...But It Works Either Way...As You Can Imagine, Use A Soft Whisper Voice Sometimes Referred To As ASMR Style.

Whispers with Me are naturally intimate
My Whispers are easily irresistible
My Whispers seem to naturally enter your mind
Easily sliding past your conscious barriers
Easily slipping into your sub-conscious
Easily sinking deeper with every word

My Whispers are naturally soothing
My Whispers are easily addicting
My Whispers are seductively enticing
Enticing you to listen
Enticing you to let go
Enticing you to go limp

My whispers are hauntingly hypnotic
My whispers are soothingly relaxing you
My whispers are softly spreading through you
Irresistibly into your mind

Irresistibly into your body
Irresistibly into your entire being

My whispers are like a sleepy drug
Dripping through your cells
My whispers are like a warm soothing blanket
Enveloping you
My whispers are like a fog
Clouding your thoughts
Compelling you to listen
Compelling you to relax
Compelling you to trance

My whisper words are intoxicatingly powerful
My whisper words are overcoming your resistance
My whisper words are becoming your world
Obeying them rapidly makes you relax deeper
Obeying them quickly makes you slide down
deeper
Obeying them obviously makes you sink further
and deeper

My Whispers.....So strong now....deeper
My Whispers.....So irresistible now....deeper
My Whispers.....So enticing now....deeper
My Whispers.....So compelling now...deeper
My Whispers.....So intimate now...Even deeper
My Whispers are.....Warm
My Whispers are.....Wonderful
My Whispers are.....Willing you down deeper
My Whispers are.....Controlling your thoughts

My Whispers are.....Compelling your mind
My Whispers are.....Commanding your obedience

With My whisper words washing through your
mind
You feel free and uninhibited
With My whisper words winding their way into
your pleasure centers
You feel your arousal...naturally building
With My whisper words waking your sexual
fantasies
You feel your wild and wanton desires flowing
Willingly giving into them
Willingly allowing the arousal
Willingly feeling the pleasure of the feelings
welling up

My whispers will you to touch yourself now
My whispers want you to feel pleasure
My whispers wind their way through you now
Wispy whispering words wandering over your body
Feel them
Wickedly naughty whispering words caressing
your mind
Give into them
Hypnotically whispering words making you feel
every touch
10 times more intense

My Whisper Trance is euphorically engaging you
In an erotically arousing fantasy flight

My Whisper Trance is making you Play and Obey
Obey and Play
My Whisper Trance is bringing your arousal to
incredible heights
Touch more intimately

My Whispers.....So strong now....pulling you
deeper...making you more aroused
The more I whisper to you...the deeper it affects
you
The deeper it affects you...the more aroused you
become
My Whispers.....So irresistible now....deeper and
closer
The more I whisper to you...the more you crave to
hear
The more you crave to hear...the more enticing it
gets
My Whispers.....So enticing now....deeper and
wanting
The more I whisper to you...the more your wanting
grows
The more the wanting grows...the more
compelling My Whispers become
My Whispers.....So compelling now...deeper and
needing to listen
The more I whisper to you...the more compelled to
listen you become
My Whispers...so arousing to you as your mind
swims in them your body reacts

The more I whisper to you...the more aroused you get

My Whispers.....So intimate now...deeper and building
My Whispers.....Warmth...becoming hotter
My Whispers.....Wonderful...becoming hotter
My Whispers.....Willing you down deeper and closer
My Whispers.....Controlling your thoughts...so aroused
My Whispers.....Compelling your mind
My Whispers.....Commanding your obedience
Whispering my command for you to Cum and Climax
Climax and cum
Play and Obey Cum
Obey and Play Climax

Exploding to My Whispers
Binds you to My Whispers
My Whispers...To Enticing To Ignore
My Whispers...Always Wanting More
My Whispers...Obey them
My Whispers...Addicting
My Whispers...Binding
My Whispers...enslaving you to the wanting
My Whispers...enslaving you to the needing
My Whispers...enslaving you to My Whisper Trances

My Whispers Always...Filling your mind...
My Whispers...From the back to the front
My Whispers...From the top to the bottom
My Whispers...From side to side

My Whispers are...Encompassing you in their
warm wrapping sounds
My Whispers are...Enchanting you in their
soothing silky seductiveness
My Whispers are...Entrancing you in their enticing
enriching ecstasy
My Whispers are...Enveloping you in their ever
entwining intimacy

Around and around...Down and down
My Whispers...Dancing and dripping over you
My Whispers...Slipping and sliding into you
My Whispers...Tugging on your mind
My Whispers...Pulling you deeper and deeper

My whisper words are again intoxicatingly
powerful
My whisper words are again overcoming your
resistance
My whisper words are again becoming your world
Obeying them rapidly makes you relax deeper
Obeying them quickly makes you slide down
deeper
Obeying them obviously makes you sink further
and deeper

My Whispers Take You Deeper now
My Whispers make you pay attention to each
word.
My Whispers make it so easy to let my words fill
your mind.
My Whispers make My every word true to you
My Whispers make My thoughts your thoughts.

My Whispers pull you in more and more.
My Whispers pulling you further and deeper into
My words.
My Whispers stronger
My Whispers deeper
My Whispers far more arousing each time...

Feel yourself being drawn into My Whispers...
Feel yourself hypnotized by My Whispers
Feel yourself so aroused by My Whispers
Feel yourself pulled ever deeper down into MY
WHISPERS
Feel yourself totally taken over by My Whispers
NOW

My Whispers make you go 10 times Deeper each
time
My Whispers make you 10 times more relaxed
each time
My Whisper waves take your mind make you
mine...
My Whisper words take you Deeper and deeper
into trance.

My Whisper words feel so good to your mind.

My Whisper words are so enticing to listen to...
My Whisper words...You can't stop listening
My Whisper words have you hypnotized.
My Whisper words have your mind and body now.
My Whisper words must be obeyed...

My Whispers make you feel so sexy and aroused
My Whispers make you want to touch yourself again
My Whispers make you think of Me when you touch
My Whispers.....So intimate now...deeper and building
My Whispers deep in your mind and surrounding your body

My Whispers.....So Warm...you're becoming sexually hotter
My Whispers.....So Wonderful...making you become so aroused again
My Whispers.....Willing you down deeper and closer...hotter
My Whispers.....Controlling your thoughts...making you so aroused
My Whispers.....Compelling your mind...to deeper sexual fantasies

My Whispers.....Commanding your obedience

My Whispers...Commanding you to get closer to a Climax again
My Whispers...Commanding you and enticing you to abandon yourself
My Whispers...Commanding you to touch and feel every nerve on edge...
My Whispers...Making you Climax and Cum

My Whispers make you feel it over, under around and through you
My Whispers make your Climax and Cum a totally new experience
My Whispers roll through you as you Cum
My Whispers capture you even tighter and deeper as you Cum
My Whispers are always in your mind now

Exploding to My Whispers again
Binds you to My Whispers again
My Whispers...To Enticing To Ignore
My Whispers...Always Wanting More
My Whispers...Obey them
My Whispers...Addicting
My Whispers...Binding
My Whispers...enslaving you to the wanting
My Whispers...enslaving you to the needing
My Whispers...enslaving you to My Whisper Trances

My Whispers Make You Want To Play This File
My Whispers Make You Want To Obey This File

My Whispers Make You Need To Play This File
My Whispers Make You Need To Obey This File
Always Wanting My Whispers From This Day On
Always Needing My Whispers From this Day On

Time To Waken To My Whispers again
But Knowing My Whispers Are Always Walking
and Wandering Through Your Mind
Waken And Remember The Wanting & Needing To
Hear My Whispers Again...The Craving Builds
Every Day
My Whispers Affect You Now In Deeper And
Deeper Ways

Waken Now On My Whisper Of Three
One Starting To Awaken And Coming Slowly Back
Two Stretching And Feeling Wonderful
Three Wide Awake...MY Whispers Are
Wonderful...Aren't They?
My Whispers are floating through you even though
you are awake.

SQUIRTING TRANCE

I'm sure you've heard the statement that, "You can't hypnotize someone against their will," haven't you? But you see, that's not exactly true...We have all yawned when we see another person doing it at one time or another...And there are muscle groups such as around your eyes and fingers that are very susceptible to suggestion

...Which is why you always hear hypnotist tell subjects that their eyes are becoming very heavy...isn't it?...Or that their fingers are stuck together when they clasp their hands tightly...But the most sensitive areas beyond your control are your erogenous zones...aren't they? You just naturally get turned on over certain things without even rationally thinking about it...It just happens...I'll bet it could be happening even now...As you imagine me taking control and stimulating your Breasts and pussy....

Just daydreaming and imagining a sexy situation like that, can really stimulate you...And naturally make it easy for me to just hypnotize that part of you...Because your sex organs have a mind of their own...don't they?...Of course they do...The human sexual drive is one of the two strongest drives we have...Sex drives can overcome anything except the will to survive...And since you're in no danger of not surviving with me...and in fact, totally enjoying this sexually stimulating experience...your minds defenses seem to automatically relax now ...And your sexual response center begins to easily weave arousing fantasies of what will happen next...And the more you relax the more arousing those fantasies will become...Even now you can feel your mind working in an erotic and arousing way...as you relax and dream...dream and think about enticing and arousing fantasies as you find yourself relaxing and giving in to those thoughts...as we count backwards to evoke even more from your mind's sexual center.

10. Even as you relax, your nipples are probably beginning to stiffen and get hard...as my words begin to weave their magic in your mind...

9. You have started finding yourself enraptured by the thoughts they are invoking...

8. My Sensual silky stroking words...Seemingly flowing to your arms and fingers...Making them move to your breasts now...As though they have a mind of their own that makes them massage, roll, pinch & pull for me...

7. The better it feels...the easier it is to give in to the feelings...isn't it?...You just naturally give in to the feelings...as they begin to overwhelm your mind with deeper and deeper pleasures...the deeper and deeper you let yourself go...

6. Your breasts and nipples are beginning to feel totally hypnotized by my words...The more you touch and play...The more they stiffen...get sensitive and arouse you... Playing and the pleasure make them want to respond even deeper.

5. Each touch, pinch, pull and caress is twice as stimulating as the last one now...And you begin to notice how totally aroused and hypnotized your breasts and nipples have become just by listening to my sensual silky words...Making you want to feel even more...

4. You feel so good now....You have no worries in the world...You do not need to even think...Just listen and respond...My thoughts will be your thoughts and you will welcome this because it will help you stay in the wonderful state of relaxation you are enjoying.....

3. You want to stay relaxed but you can only do so if you read (Listen to) my words and obey all my instructions...You do not wish to resist my words because if you do you know you will no longer be relaxed and you want to avoid that at all costs.

2. Tell me in your mind...that you love this ...that's right...As you say it my words arouse you even more...Now just let you minds sexual center hook all three areas together... Your breasts & nipples and your pussy & clit...

1. Feel the neural pathways open and link them...so that even just flicking your nipple with a fingertip feels like you are flicking the tip of your Clit. Your pussy and Nipples are becoming one...Tripling the arousal and the pleasure sensations assaulting your mind...and making your body respond three times greater to my words...

NOW...as we begin to move down...down...down and hypnotize your pelvis area...from front to back and inside and out...Deeper and deeper...Every nerve ending is becoming totally alive and aroused for me...Responding to my words and thoughts floating into your mind and shooting down your spine...pulling you down...Down into My Silky sensual hypnotic words Your pussy lips swollen and silky with moisture...as one arm...hand...and fingers are playing with your pussy ...and making your clit harden even more than it already is...You can feel the wetness flowing...drenching you...drift down... pulling your mind down to focus on the dreamy dripping creamy arousal that is building around your swollen Clit...

The first touch is almost electric...shooting sensations to your mind... amplified on my words ...And as you roll a nipple and your clit at the same time...You feel the neural connection enhanced and doubled...Now sliding over to the other nipple to enhance and double that connection...That's right...

Falling & Floating...
You've begun to Fall Deeper
Slowly & Gently...
Over Around & Through
Deeply & Directly, Drifting & Dreamy
Focus & Fall...Aroused and Wet
Follow My Words
Obey Your Desires
Drowsy & Drifting
Slipping & Sliding Down
You've begun to Fall Deeply
Falling and Floating

Faster and Deeper
Deeply Drifting
Drifting & Dreaming
Floating & Falling
Focus & Fall Deeper
Nothing Else Matters
Drowsy & Horny
Drifting
Slipping
Sliding

Deeper
Focused On My Words
Slip Deeper
Fall Deeper
Drift Deeper
Float Deeper
Always Deeper
Loving My Words
Slipping Deeper
Fingers sliding in finding your G-spot
Slipping over it...Rubbing it and loving the sensations
Falling deeper into the arousal with each touch
Slipping & Sliding...Floating on the sensations
Always Sliding Deeper
Sliding your middle FINGER DEEPER...Your finger Sliding deep inside, now finding your deep spot...The deeper they slide...the wetter and more aroused you get...And the more aroused you get...the deeper hypnotized your breasts and

pussy get...As you slide your finger around and over your deep spot...you may feel like it is making you feel similar to the urge to pee...but this is actually the naturally building of your ejaculate getting ready to squirt when you cum

In fact you are now finding that your whole mind and body is becoming totally aroused...And because your whole self is feeling it...Your whole self just naturally slips deeply into hypnosis for me...Slipping down on the arousal and touches...Sliding ever deeper as you come ever closer to going over the edge and climaxing as my words take you deeper and closer...closer and deeper...Slipping and falling...sliding down as your fingers slide deeper and then out over and around your clit...Feel the dizzying effects of your total arousal in your mind and body...The swirling sensations of pleasure building and building...taking you ever closer to an amazing hot squirting climax that you can no longer stop from happening...Hung on my every hypnotic word now as you hover on the edge...loving every second...knowing what is coming now...Touching faster and deeper...deeper and faster ...closer...closer...closer..NOW CUM...CUM AND CLIMAX FOR ME... CUM HARD...DEEP...LET THE WAVES OF PLEASURE ROLL OVER... UNDER AROUND AND THROUGH YOU...REVERBERATING IN YOUR MIND...LOCKING YOUR MIND ON YOUR SQUIRTING...REVELLING IN THE FEELINGS... AS

THEY LAP AT YOUR MIND IN WAVE AFTER WAVE OF INCREDIBLE PLEASURE...

Now even as the INCREDIBLE WAVES OF PLEASURE slowly subside ...your conscious mind begins to realize just how powerful my hypnotic suggestions still are...And begins to craft hypnotic words, suggestions and ideas for you to use ON YOURSELF...SIMPLY BY USING OUR BLUEROSE WORD TO TAKE YOU BACK HERE WHENEVER YOU CHOOSE...

NOW I WANT YOU TO CLOSE YOUR EYES AND SLOWLY COUNT UP FROM ONE TO FIVE IN YOU MIND...WITH EACH COUNT YOU WILL REALIZE HOW INCREDIBLE MY WORDS HAVE BEEN TO YOU...AND ON FIVE YOU'LL AWAKEN FEELING SO WONDERFUL YOU'LL NATURALLY WANT MORE...Begin to count now...

SEXTRANCE DOMME INDUCTION

In this instance...You take total control right from the beginning. It has multiple "sexual hypnotic anchors" built in.

For the mp3 you need to do some instructions in the beginning:

HYPNOTEUSE: Get ready for a journey with me...Find a nice...comfortable ...private place to

listen...Perhaps even your bedroom...I'd like to be in your bedroom with you...Watching you respond to my voice...my image in your mind...

HYPNOTEUSE: You seem to be interested in me...aren't you?

SUBJECT: Yes (naturally...lol)

HYPNOTEUSE: But, I'm only interested in men who submit to my sexual hypnotic control...You can deal with that if you want me...can't you?

SUBJECT: Yes.

HYPNOTEUSE: Good...Because you interest me...and I know you'll enjoy what I will do to you....won't you?

SUBJECT: Yes.

HYPNOTEUSE: In fact...You find yourself already aroused at the thought of my sexual hypnotic control...aren't you?

SUBJECT: Yes.

HYPNOTEUSE: Good...That arouses my interest in continuing with you. A funny thing arousal...Such a strong primitive emotion...Something you can't stop or fight...Just like my trances...In fact they are linked in your mind now...Arousal...My hypnotic trances...All one...Because the more aroused you become with me...the easier it is to slip into my trance. Just picture my naked body in your mind...I know you can do that easily...can't you?

SUBJECT: Yes

HYPNOTEUSE: Excellent...Now as your eyes run over every inch...you can feel each corresponding part of your body relax for me...Start with my feet...Imagine my toes...painted...sparkling in your eyes...And feel Your toes relax and let go, as mine wiggle and capture the gaze in your minds eye (You can do this for real "one on one"...I'm assuming it is over the "net") The muscle power disappears from yours...they go limp and relaxed...Feel my mind in yours...Pulling the tension away...Now let your imaginary gaze fall upon my ankles...See them rotate...as yours relax...and totally let go...You feel your ankles getting loose and limp...letting go for me...don't you?

SUBJECT: Yes

HYPNOTEUSE: Good...You are doing well...Let your gaze flow up my smooth calf...so inviting...so promising...strong...taking the muscle power from yours...Your calves now letting go...It feels so incredible...Let it happen...It arouses me to imagine your muscles respond to my suggestions...And arouses you more...seeing my arousal in your mind...Now look at my knees...slightly bent...soft and inviting...let yours go...become soft and limp...And follow up my thighs...Drawing you to the place you want so much...taking all your tension from your thighs...letting them go limp and relaxed...Now concentrate on my hips and vagina...Since you don't have a vagina...(If you are working with a

woman...this would change to making her as aroused as you are.)...Your penis will not relax...it will get even harder...as you imagine the glistening silkiness of my pussy lips sparkle and capture your mind's pleasure center...So wet...So inviting...Making you so hard...but feeling your hips let go...As you totally concentrate on my pussy...you lower and upper back muscles totally relax...You can't fight the hypnotic sexual power of my mind and pussy...you are finding you don't want to...It feels too good...too arousing to do as I suggest...to let yourself go for me...doesn't it?

SUBJECT: Yes.

HYPNOTEUSE: Yes...So good...as you let your shoulders slump...and take your gaze up for a minute...to my gorgeous breasts...Imagine them...nipples stiff and erect for you...As they drain all the muscle power from your chest...Feel yourself completely sinking into the soft comfortable place for me...Even your stomach and abdomen limp loose and relaxed now...Turning over control to me feels incredible...It makes you more aroused than you have ever been in your life...Watch as you relax your arms and hands for me...Your penis (or clit for a woman) gets rock hard...Let your arms loose...shoulders to elbows... elbows all the way out your fingertips...Now be aware of how hard you are...from turning control over to me...How turned on this submission to my trance has made you...And will always make you...Now imagine your gaze falling on my face...Locking onto my deep (your color) eyes...As your head, neck, and facial muscles relax...Feel yourself falling into them...ever so deeper as I count backwards from 10 to 0. 10...falling deep...opening your mind to me...relaxing all defenses...letting me in...9...totally letting your control go...letting my control permeate you...8...Feel yourself submitting to my every wish...and getting unbelievable pleasure from it..7...Feel me at the depths of your mind...taking control...6...feel the last resistance fade...your mind totally opening to me now...5...Feel the incredible arousal this submission to my will brings you...You have never felt such pleasure...and it will increase even more...as you let yourself fall deeper into my control...4...Your entire sexual pleasure center opening to me...to my suggestions...3...Your body responding only to my suggestions now...as you feel your excitement and arousal grow as I take over...2...You are very close to an orgasm now...feel the throbbing...feel the pressure building...I will make it happen automatically ...when I say zero...you will find that I control your orgasms now...you will cum for me...harder and deeper than at any time in your life...1...This hypnotic climax will cement my suggestions in your mind...You will feel my vagina around your penis in your mind...pulling...taking you in...riding your hardness and not letting you stop...feel it now...building...cementing my control...and as you cum...a lock snaps in place in you mind...It will be there for me to unlock whenever I wish...to enter and control by simply saying the words (Your favorite trigger) to you...your cock will stiffen...and your mind will open to my control...You WILL BE MY TOTAL SEXUAL HYPNOTIC SLAVE WHEN YOU CLIMAX...And you are too close to stop it...0...Cum for me...0...Cement my control in your mind...0...My sexual hypnotic slave forever...0...so powerful...as only I can make your climaxes for you...Yes...feel it my hypnotic sex slave...your mind so weak now...just feeling so...good... slipping deeper into my total control... you love to please me with your climaxes...to shower yourself in wet cum for me...makes you want to please me...you can feel yourself slipping deeper now...slip...deeper for me...slide down totally...to the place where I control your thoughts...my sleepy hypnotic pet...where I command and you obey...feel your arousal again...following my commands arouses you...makes you weak...you find yourself following my every word now...aroused and relaxed...wanting to be with me...to please me...I know what is good for you....what you need...and you know what I need...I am your mistress...you want to take care of me...to fulfill my needs...deeper now pet...fulfilling my needs is so important to you now...You know it is...deep in your mind now...cemented there with unbreakable bonds... mental bonds...wrapping around you now..

arousing bonds...pleasing me makes them stronger...you so want to please me now...in every way...when you awaken...as soon as you can contact me...you will...and you will find yourself wanting to please me in any way I request...it is so important to you...and the more you listen to my voice...the deeper you will go...and the deeper you go...the more you will please me...you must please your Mistress...pleasing me...brings pleasure to you my weak hypnotic pet...feel your arousal build as you crave to please me...to do as I ask...deeper and more aroused...cemented and bonded to me...feeling my lovely hypnotic bonds slipping around you...penetrating the deepest portions of your mind...feel me tug on them... bringing you closer...you cannot resist now...they are too strong...resisting me in any way simply strengthens them...trying to resist makes you weaker...the more you resist me...the deeper my control becomes...and the more you find yourself wanting my control...in every way...every day...deeper...every way deeper...please me my hypnotic pet...shower me with your submission ...deeper now...spiraling into my hypnotic depths...

COCOON INDUCTION

You've seen a cocoon at sometime in your life... haven't you?

And I'll bet you can imagine one for me NOW...can't you? (If this were "live" one on one, you would ask them to close their eyes, just listen and imagine.)

Imagine the silvery strands glistening in the light...Spinning and weaving around and around...

NOTICE how the Strands seem to capture your attention...So many to FOLLOW...MY lovely WEB IS so FACINATING to YOU..NOW

SPINNING around and around...DOWN and down...towards the center...So BEAUTIFUL to look at...FACINATING and CAPTIVATING to your mind...isn't it?

Yes...MY WEB IS so very ENTICING AND SENSUAL to you NOW...MY WEB OF WORDS is like A COCOON...WRAPPING AROUND YOU NOW...

Softly encasing your mind in silvery strands...Around and around...Deeper and deeper...

You see how easily YOU FOLLOW my lines...Don't you?

Yes...And you do want ME to continue...don't you?

Good...YOU can almost FEEL your mind spinning down towards the center...towards ME..can't you?

Yes...My words TAKING YOU there...Do this for me NOW...
Imagine a circle of MY SILKY SENSUAL STRANDS WRAPPING AROUND YOUR MIND NOW...Your inner self stands on the edge of the first line...YOU can see yourself there...Can't you?

Yes...Very Nice...You FOLLOW it like you follow MY WORDS...Around and around...TAKING YOU DOWN and DOWN...

DEEPER and DEEPER towards the center...YOU ARE WITHIN MY CIRCLE OF WORDS AND STRANDS NOW...You can see that...Can't you?

Yes...You are doing so well...YOU can see in your mind NOW...GO DEEPER into the circle...ALL THE WAY DOWN at the very center shrouded in mist is me...You do want to SEE ME NOW...don't you?

YES...of course you do...It excites you to THINK OF ME THERE NOW...doesn't it?

Yes...it does...You would like to COME TO ME THERE NOW...To be TOTALLY WRAPPED IN MY SENSUAL SILKEN STRANDS...wouldn't you?

Yes...I knew you would...THEN COME TO ME NOW...Round and round...Deeper and deeper down...So relaxing and arousing to TOTALLY LET GO FOR ME NOW...SO DEEP...SLIPPING DEEPER into my sensual web...SLIDING DOWN...LETTING GO...FREEFALLING towards me...ALL CONTROL SLIPPING AWAY...You FEEL MY MENTAL PULL growing stronger...Don't you?

Yes...ENVELOPING YOU...as your RESISTANCE MELTS AWAY...You FEEL YOURSELF TURNING CONTROL OVER TO ME...It's so IRRESTIBLE...so INVITING...so EXCITING...AND so AROUSING NOW...You feel YOUR WILL SLIPPING AWAY...MY WILL WRAPPING AROUND YOUR MIND NOW...MY SILVERY STRANDS TAKING CONTROL...as you COME CLOSER...And the closer you GET the MORE SEXUALLY EXCITED you grow...

You can almost SEE ME NOW...You CRAVE TO SEE ME NOW...NEED TO SEE ME NOW...The need grows and grows...doesn't it?

YES..COME TO ME NOW...COME CLOSER...GO DEEPER...CLOSER...DEEPER...You can SEE ME NOW...A SHIMMERING SENSUAL SILOUETTE...TANTALIZING YOU...INVITING YOU DEEPER NOW...Come closer...GO DEEPER...You so want to COME CLOSER and GO DEEPER...don't you?

Yes...I knew YOU would...Now FEEL the SILKY STRANDS of my web SPIN OUT FROM ME...and TOUCH YOUR SKIN...SO SOFT...SO SENSUALLY AROUSING...The more strands that touch you...the DEEPER you go NOW...And the DEEPER you go...the MORE AROUSED you get...

YOU NEED TO GO DEEPER NOW...EACH WORD SENDS YOU DEEPER...EACH AROUSING STRAND SENDS YOU DEEPER...YOU CRAVE TO BE TOTALLY ENVELOPED IN ME...don't you? (This next part is only for typed inductions...skip it for voice or in person.)

Yes...And YOU WILL BE...In just a minute when you see the word ENVELOPED again...I want you to close your eyes and imagine yourself FALLING TO ME IN THE VERY CENTER OF MY WEB...FALLING SO DEEPLY...TOTALLY ENTRANCED IN MY AROUSING PRESENCE...When you reach me and FEEL MY WEB CLOSE AROUND YOU...open your eyes and type "Totally Enveloped" back to me...You will do this for me...won't you?

Good...So good to be ENVELOPED!

(Wait for them to type "Totally Entranced", then continue. Here is where you would pick up on a live or voice induction.)

Yes...MY PET...FEEL MY WEB TOTALLY AROUND YOU AND SEEPING THROUGH YOUR SKIN NOW...ENVELOPING...AROUSING...SURROUNDING YOUR MIND...PENETRATING IT DO THE DEEPEST CORE...Like the SOFT SILKEN CARESSES of my words...My strands TOUCH YOU EVERYWHERE...STIMULATING YOUR SEXUAL CENTERS...and at the same time...ENVELOPING YOUR CONSCIOUS MIND...STRAND AFTER STRAND...AROUND AND AROUND...DEEPER AND DEEPER...COOCONED AND CONTROLLED BY MY STRANDS...FILLED WITH MIND NUMBING SECRETIONS...EACH STRAND DRIPS AWAY NOW...EACH DROP PENETRATES...YOUR LAST CONTROL...FALLING AWAY NOW...FALLING DEEPER INTO MY CONTROL...YOUR WILL TO RESIST ME...GONE... DRIP...DRIP...DRIP...YOUR MUSCLE CONTROL..GONE... DRIP...DRIP...DRIP... SURRENDERING TOTALLY TO ME...I CONTROL YOUR MIND NOW...YOUR BODY NOW...Don't I my Pet?

(A yes here, means you can pretty much do what you want with them. so go play and have fun. Take them through their "senses" and anchor every one to you...Including their "Sixth Sense".)

Feel how IT EXCITES YOU...Excites you TO SUBMIT to the pleasure of the excitement TOTALLY...The DEEPER you feel it the more YOU SUBMIT TO it...With a vision of ME DEEP IN YOUR

MIND...Let this word NOW become an invisible tattoo that you only see with me. ETCHED now on your wrist...PERMANENTLY...and....DEEPLY in your skin...And whenever I tell you to touch it...you will come back to me in this place NOW and forever...When you touch it...It make you THINK OF ME...EACH TIME YOU TOUCH IT... YOU DO understand and OBEY THIS...don't you?
Yes
Of course you do...there is so much PLEASURE in touching NOW in your wrist...It is now ADDICTING YOU...TO ME...That is a fun ADDICTION that GROWS WHEN YOU TOUCH "NOW"...So DEEP an ADDICTION FOR ME...that ADDICTS YOU NOW...and LOCKS DEEPLY IN YOUR MIND... doesn't it?
Yes

You know that NOW you will also SEE EROTIC IMAGES OF ME IN YOUR MIND...They're AROUSING and SENSUOUSLY STIMULATING... CAPTIVATING your SEXUAL response...NOW...all beautiful things YOU SEE...take your mind back to ME...Hovering OVER YOU in your mind...

CONTROLING your passion....YOU...so responsive to MY IMAGE IN YOUR MIND...THINKING OF ME MAKES YOU AROUSED...NOW...and ALWAYS brings you pleasure DEEPER in your mind....IN MY WORDS there is ALWAYS happiness...making you SO CONTENT...So wonderful to LET GO OF YOUR

WILL...BECOME OBEDIENT TO THE SIGHT OF ME...You will LET GO TOTALLY...NOW...won't you?
Yes
That SOUNDS wonderful to me NOW...I'd love you to hear me...AROUSE YOU...with the SOUND OF ONLY MY VOICE...It BRINGS YOU EXSTACY with DEEPER sounds NOW...MY VOICE FILLS YOUR MIND...INVADES YOUR BEING...The BINDING melodies that bring YOU TO ME...Dancing and SWIRLING...BUILDING UNBREAKABLE BONDS...SUBMITTING your ears to the most pleasant sounds...TO ME...MY MUSICAL VOICE is SO CAPTIVATING...Even YOU CAN"T RESIST IT AS YOU HEAR MY WORDS IN YOUR MIND...NOW...Can you?
No
No...I know you couldn't....By NOW...you want me so much...You can almost TASTE ME...Feel the wanting building NOW...as you LICK YOUR WRIST...and IMAGINE IT IS ME...The wonderfully EROTIC ESSENCE OF ME...You can DO IT NOW...LICK AND CARESS your wrist for ME....FEEL ME RESPOND in your mind...INTOXICATING your taste buds and BUILDING our bonds ever so STRONGER WITH EACH TASTE OF ME ON YOUR WRIST...IMAGINE MY ESSENCE...MY SEX...MY PHRENOMES INVADING YOUR MIND...THE TASTE LIKE THE SWEETEST THING YOU COULD IMAGINE...Mingling with YOUR TASTE...Just because you are UNDER MY CONTROL... CRAVING

MY TASTE....So that from NOW on FAVORITE FOODS WILL TASTE LIKE ME...Won't they?

Yes

Yes...my sweet ONE....NOW EVEN the SMELL of things REMINDS YOU OF ME...Breathe in MY CAPTIVATING ESSENCE...See...It SWIMS IN...IN YOUR SOUL...CAPTURING...AROUSING YOU TOTALLY... It Is PERVADING all your NERVE ENDINGS...NOW...with the sweet smell of TOTAL SURRENDER TO ME...Waves of EROTIC PLEASURES AWAIT YOU. You know that IF YOU TOTALLY SURRENDER TO MY CONTROL...Your mind will FOLLOW WHAT I SAY WITHOUT QUESTION...And YOUR REWARDYOU'RE YOUR SURRENDER IS only a short distance away...It could be ORGASMIC BLISS in the short term...AND TOTAL SUBMISSION TO ME when you surrender yourself. You feel the pressure of the ORGASMIC BLISS OF SURRENDER coursing through you...It is COMING FROM ME...NOW...Making you want to ASK ME for RELEASE...isn't it?

Yes...PLEASE

NOW TO THE FINAL PHASE OF TYING IN EMOTIONS:

That's a nice "please" for NOW...but I don't FEEL it in YOUR EMOTIONS I don't FEEL YOUR WANTING ME IN YOUR SOUL...I think you FEEL IT IN YOUR TASTE NOW...AND FEEL ME IN YOUR SMELL NOW...And SEE AND HEAR ME IN YOUR MIND

NOW...And perhaps even **FEEL MY TOUCH NOW...But...NOW...FEEL YOUR TOTAL ADORATION FOR ME...TAKING YOU OVER....**Isn't it?

Yes

Yes...**NOW TOTALLY AROUSED BY MY PRESENCE...**You would be **SO SAD IF I LEFT YOU...YOU CAN IMAGINE THAT NOW...SADNESS, LONELINESS, EMPTYNESS WITHOUT ME...NOW ...FEEL THAT...YOU HATE THE THOUGHT...**don't you?

Yes

TELL ME HOW YOU WOULD FEEL...MAKE ME WANT TO STAY...TO GIVE YOU WHAT YOU WANT....TELL ME NOW...

(Wait for answer...And make them get really involved in it. Become their "Master or Goddess".)

Good Love....**NOW** I am happy to know you better...To **KNOW HOW MUCH YOU LOVE AND ADORE MY PRESENCE...**I want you to **BE ESTATICALLY HAPPY AROUND ME...**Can you **FEEL THAT HAPPINESS** in my presence? **FEEL THE JOY OF SURRENDER TO ME...LOVE THE AROUSAL OF MY WORDS...NOW?**

Yes

NOW...FEEL THAT AROUSAL BUILD

USE YOUR FAVORITE SUGGESTIONS TO TAKE THEM TO A MINDBLOWING CLIMAX BUT JUST AS THEY ARE ON THE VERGE DO THIS:

SO CLOSE NOW...SO CRAVING ME NOW....SO CRAVING MY RELEASE NOW...THAT WHEN I LET YOU RELEASE FOR ME NOW....MY HYPNOTIC WEB OF CLIMAXC CLOSES OVER YOU...BINDING YOU TO ME FOREVER NOW...MY HYPNOTIC STRANDS ENVELOPE YOUR MIND SO STRONGLY NOW...THAT THE WORD "ENVELOPED" FOLLOWED BY ANY WORD I CHOOSE IS INSTANTLY ACTED UPON BY YOUR SUBCONSCIOUS...NO HESITATION NOW...

NO RESISTANCE NOW...TOTALLY MINE NOW...AS YOU FEEL YOURSELF GETTING READY TO EXPLODE NOW...CEMENTING OUR BONDS NOW... AS YOU RELEASE...NOW AND EXPLODE TO THE UNIVERSE FOR ME...NOW...NOTHING CAN STOP IT NOW...EXPLODE AND CUM...

WHEN THEY HAVE FINISHED, DO THIS:

NOW SLEEP FOR ME...KNOWING THAT FROM NOW ON UNDER HYPNOSIS...OR AWAKE...YOUR ARE NOW MINE...AND THE WORD "ENVELOPED" IS MY BINDING COMMAND ON YOU FROM NOW ON..IN THE HERE AND NOW...THE FUTURE NOW...THE FOREVER NOW...AND ENDLESS CIRCLE NOW...AND ALWAYS INTO NOW...

AWAKEN, BUT THEN THROW THE "NOW" TRIGGER AT THEM WITHIN A MINUTE AFTER

AWAKENING TO REINFORCE IT....YOU "NOW" HAVE A TRAINED SUBJECT...

ENTANGLED

According to all the new theories of Entanglement, sub atomic particles can exist in two places at one time...and vibrate together at the same frequency once they come close enough...

How interesting to think that my particles could be in your mind right now...Just think about that...Swirling around slipping ever deeper...Vibrating and resonating within you...

Weaving their magic...Just flowing everywhere ...Surrounding and entwining your thought processes...dampening them...So that you can simply relax to my words as they continue to entangle and entwine around your neurons and thoughts...

Let them...Give up and give in to them as they vibrate to your frequencies matching and humming in your mind until you don't want it to stop...It feels too nice...It's too enticing...

No Don't fight it...it is so much easier to let the vibrations match yours...Yes...like that feeling the soothing warmth of the entanglement...Pulling you closer...drifting in it. Loving the feeling...as you drop deeper with every vibrating word now.

I'll bet you can feel them deeper now...slipping and sliding through your senses one by one...Vocally first as my voice seems to drive deeper into your mind telling you to give up to it...to give in totally to it...(Repeat)

Like sweet music to your submissive impulses...My irresistible deep voice snaking it's way even deeper into your mind...Wrapping it's coils and smooth seductive power around you...Squeezing out any and all resistance you had just moments ago...Seducing you deeper...Taking you down into that warm well of trance...Deeper and further...Further and deeper...

As you follow it further and deeper...You begin to blink...and go blank...each blink making you want to close your eyes so that you can see the images in your minds eye...Your sight feels it...and now sees my deep brown eyes boring ever deeper into your core...blinking and closing now in blank obedience...

Seeing how easily they reach into your depths and find that longing to fall even deeper...Imagine riding them like laser beams of seductive sensual light...bathing your sexual center in hot flashes...Causing it to respond with arousal...So easily and naturally that you know the feelings are multiplying with each passing second

Falling deeper as they well up and spread from atom to atom...cell to cell...nerve ending to nerve ending...Cascading and feeding off my voice and my eyes...So nice to let go and give into it...The more you let go now...the deeper you drift...And the deeper you drift the more sexual excitement you feel...

And as you breathe deeply for me...You begin to catch a whiff or your own arousal wafting up from between your legs...Causing the arousal to double as your wetness starts to flow...And the scent starts to increase...It's easy now to imagine my seductive scent mingling with yours...

Breathe them in...let them flow through you...Let them arouse totally...With every breath you take deeper down and more aroused. Dropping you into that warm well of sexual arousal and compliance...The deeper you go the more alive your arousal seems to become.

Growing and connecting every nerve ending together...Feel it spreading now over under around and through you...The scent of sex is overwhelming...and building making you want to remove your clothing...to inhale the scents as you bring your moist panties closer to your face...and breathe in...Giving in to the arousal of the scents...The exotic and erotic essences of your own wetness...

It seems to make you want to taste your hot wet juices now...To mingle touch with taste...No control now...You simply find your fingers flowing down...flying to your warm wet throbbing pussy...pulling you deeper as they do...

Touching...caressing rubbing and tasting yourself...The more you touch...the more alive with sexual energy all the particles that have migrated everywhere seem to be...My particles entangled with yours...

Moving into you even now...Controlling you now... Encouraging you now...Making your wet fingers of one hand trail up your body and around your stiff nipples...As you roll and pinch them...they send sparks through the particles and deeper into your minds sexual center...Sending the arousal back through every nerve ending at lightning speed....Shooting your fingers on the other hand to your throbbing clit... as the other continues playing with your aroused nipples and breasts...Feeling your hips raise to each touch now...The more you touch...the more intense the arousal gets...Even your ass wants attention... leaning over to one side so you can slap it and feel the increasing intense pleasure you feel from my words and you own mind pulling you ever deeper into this hot and haunting sex trance...

You can feel the urge to take the hand from your breast and wet your fingers in your mouth...sliding then along the slit in your ass...rimming your anus...maybe even sliding in...as you work the other hand inside your wet hot pussy...deeper and warmer...slipping in and out ...over and around...so sexy to feel fingers inside both places...playing and obeying every one of my words....Because we are now totally entangled...entwined... bodies and minds...with the enhanced sexual energy of two bodies feeling like one.

My mind touching your mind...seems to enhance your responses in every way you've ever dreamed of...As though every touch is from me...Enhancing every response...increasing every pleasure sensation...Reaching places in your minds sexual center even you had not known about...

Stimulating them as I increase our sexual vibrations...Feel it now...Love it now...Losing yourself in it now...There is no way to stop this now...You simply find now that the arousal and feelings are building like a tidal wave...The more you touch for me...the deeper you go for me...And the deeper you go the closer you get to exploding for me...The well of trance is so deep now...The tidal wave of arousal so strong...Coming closer and falling deeper...Imagining me in you now...in every opening...every cell...whispering CUM FOR ME NOW...CUM HARD AND DEEP...LET THE TIDAL WAVE BREAK OVER YOU NOW...SWIRLING YOU IN A GIANT CLIMAX...THAT'S RIGHT GIVE IT ALL...FEEL IT ALL...A TOTAL MIND AND BODY CLIMAX...THAT REVERBERATES THROUGH YOU...INTO EVERY PARTICLE OF OUR BEINGS...BLENDING AND ENTWINING US IN UNBREAKABLE PARTICLE BONDS...AS EVERY WAVE ASSAULTS YOUR MIND AND BODY...LIKE FIREWORKS GOING OFF N A SPECTACULAR CRESCENDO OF CLIMAXES

Now as you slowly feel the first climax subside into aftershocks...you feel each one with incredible pleasure...as you drift on the feelings and flow even deeper... until you are ready to come back and slowly count from one to five so alive...so satisfied...so warm and fuzzy when you reach five and awaken totally...Wanting to experience even more...

END

CLOSING STATEMENT:

I hope you continue to enjoy "Hypnosis For Lovers", and we will keep you in mind for our future "Advanced Seminars" coming out in late 2017 and early 2018..If you would like information on Seminars or the Audio Version of this course, please E-Mail hypnoventures@yahoo.com

HYPNOTICALLY,

Richard Anthony,
"HYPNOSIS FOR LOVERS" Author